Legends

and

Legacies

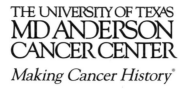

THE UNIVERSITY OF TEXAS
MD ANDERSON
CANCER CENTER
Making Cancer History®

Elizabeth L. Travis, Ph.D., is Associate Vice President for Women Faculty
Programs, Professor of Experimental Radiation Oncology
and Mattie Allen Fair Professor in Cancer Research at
The University of Texas M. D. Anderson Cancer Center.

ISBN 978-0-9753878-1-8

FIRST EDITION

Produced by M. D. Anderson's offices:
Women Faculty Programs, Public Affairs and Scientific Publications

Editor: Elizabeth L. Travis, Ph.D.
Jacket and book design: Maria E. Dungler
Group photos: John Smallwood and Ray Garcia
Photo editing: Kelley Moore
Cover stock images: ©iStockphoto

Published in Houston, Texas, U.S.A.
October 2008

Table of Contents

FOREWORD
John Mendelsohn, M.D.
President and Professor of Cancer Medicine
The University of Texas M. D. Anderson Cancer Center

PREFACE
Elizabeth L. Travis, Ph.D.
Associate Vice President for Women Faculty Programs
Professor of Experimental Radiation Oncology
Mattie Allen Fair Professor in Cancer Research
The University of Texas M. D. Anderson Cancer Center

CHAPTERS

Table of Contents

Table of Contents

EPILOGUE
Raymond N. DuBois, M.D., Ph.D.
Provost and Executive Vice President
Professor of Gastrointestinal Medical Oncology
The University of Texas M. D. Anderson Cancer Center

Foreword

Long before I became President of M. D. Anderson in 1996, I was well aware of the many talented physicians and scientists whose contributions had helped develop this institution as an international leader in research-driven cancer patient care. As I have learned much more about the remarkable history and the pioneers who left powerful footprints for us to follow, I have been increasingly impressed by the number of women faculty so critical to the progress on which we are building today.

Legends and Legacies is a captivating collection of the personal journeys taken by 26 of our successful women physicians and scientists. After reading their stories, I was struck by how diverse — and often difficult — their pilgrimages have been, yet all share the common bond of growing up knowing they wanted to make a difference. Some were the first in their families to attend college, while others are carrying on scientific traditions inspired by parents and grandparents who were health care professionals. A few thought they would be teachers, one aspired to become a dancer, and another originally planned to be a nuclear physicist. Several recall expecting to escape childhood hardships, including one whose parents were migrant farm workers. Even those with extremely limited economic means remember being encouraged by mothers and fathers to get an education. Their cumulative roots represent a rich smorgasbord of cultures, from India, Japan, South Africa, Mexico, China and Canada as well as a cross section of American small towns and large cities.

An influential thread uniting these women involves how they overcame the unfortunate discrimination that has existed far too long against those who strived for careers in the biomedical sciences. Some tell how they also had to tolerate racial and social biases on top of the gender issues. Central to each journey is the innate tenacity to succeed combined with the importance of caring mentors, both men and women, who during different periods had a profound impact on their career development. Most describe their dilemmas concerning how they could balance marriage — plus if and when to have children — with demanding responsibilities at a major academic institution. The women whose husbands also are physicians and scientists discuss the tough choices they faced in deciding to come to M. D. Anderson. Nearly all of the stories include details of how these women learned organizational and leadership skills needed to advance into key administrative positions and accept important assignments that provide national visibility. Most offer insights about how they have achieved harmony in their professional and personal lives.

M. D. Anderson has a long-standing interest in expanding opportunities for its women faculty. Margaret L. Kripke, Ph.D., who in 1983 was named the first woman to chair a department (Immunology), raised concerns about equitable recruitment, salary and promotion while serving as the inaugural chair of the Committee on the Status of Women and Minorities as well as founding chair of the Women's Faculty Organization. She also achieved many other "firsts," including the first woman faculty member selected to top management. Even though she retired in 2007 as our Executive Vice President and Chief Academic Officer, she has continued to inspire us all with her unwavering advocacy for women in medicine and science. Her legacy will live on through the Office of Women Faculty Programs, which we established to coordinate myriad activities aimed at identifying and implementing career development options for women faculty, promoting networking and mentoring, and advising senior leaders about important issues as well as women who should be considered for leadership positions.

I am grateful to Elizabeth L. Travis, Ph.D., our first Associate Vice President for Women Faculty Programs, for leading our efforts to make M. D. Anderson the number one destination for women physicians and scientists in cancer-focused patient care, research, education and prevention. She has led development of *Legends and Legacies*, which I believe all readers will find fascinating.

John Mendelsohn, M.D.
President and Professor of Cancer Medicine
The University of Texas M. D. Anderson Cancer Center

Preface

This book celebrates the stellar successes of 26 women physicians and scientists who share their stories of productive careers at M. D. Anderson Cancer Center. Collectively, they represent the very best of our many talented faculty who are providing state-of-the-art patient care, helping teach the next generation of health care professionals and conducting cutting-edge research that is reducing the impact of cancer for people throughout the world.

As a faculty member at M. D. Anderson for 25 years, I have had the pleasure of working with most of the women who chronicle their journeys in *Legends and Legacies*. When I was appointed the first Associate Vice President for Women Faculty Programs in 2006, one of my early goals was to recognize the impressive — and increasing — accomplishments of all our women faculty while enhancing advocacy efforts that will improve opportunities for women at our institution as well as in our numerous professional societies. Another mutual goal for all of us in leadership positions involves inspiring young women to enter the biomedical sciences. Certainly, I am pleased that this book honors some of our women faculty, and in doing so I am excited about how it, hopefully, will motivate high school and college students to consider careers in medicine and science.

The most difficult part of planning this book was selecting the contributors because we have so many women faculty from diverse backgrounds with interesting stories to tell. Our diversity is illustrated through our professional roles, ranging from clinicians who diagnose and treat all forms of cancer, physician-scientists who apply findings from laboratory research to improve therapies, basic scientists who make the discoveries that unlock cancer-related mysteries, faculty who focus on preventing cancer by identifying individuals at high risk and/or offering programs to change behaviors, and veterinarians who coordinate the care and use of animals critical to new knowledge about cancer. The individual stories provide uniquely personal descriptions of the triumphs, failures and disappointments that we have faced while developing our careers. The common thread that connects us is our passion for helping others while balancing our professional lives with enjoying our families.

Although about 50 percent of medical school graduates and Ph.D. degrees in the life sciences are now awarded to women, the proportion of women in related careers at academic institutions across the country is woefully under-represented, particularly in the full professor and executive ranks. M. D. Anderson has a long-standing interest in recruiting and promoting women, yet only about one-third of our faculty are women.

The over-arching objective for the Office of Women Faculty Programs is for M. D. Anderson to become the number one destination for women physicians and scientists in cancer treatment and research. I am optimistic that this book will help us realize that vision.

I want to thank Diane Hackett for copyediting this book, Mary Jane Schier for her expertise and editorial assistance, Maria Dungler for the book design and her staff (Kelley Moore, Gini Reed, Eli Gukich and Erin McCormick) for their creative contributions, photographer John Smallwood, and especially Ray DuBois for his encouragement and enthusiastic support of *Legends and Legacies*. Finally, I will always be grateful to my friends and colleagues who so willingly shared their wonderful stories.

Elizabeth L. Travis, Ph.D.
Associate Vice President for Women Faculty Programs
Professor of Experimental Radiation Oncology
Mattie Allen Fair Professor in Cancer Research
The University of Texas M. D. Anderson Cancer Center

Janet M. Bruner, M. D.

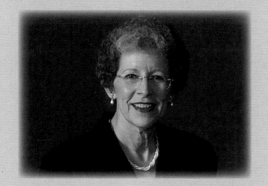

Professor and Chair of Pathology
Ferenc and Phyllis Gyorkey Chair
for Research and Education in Pathology

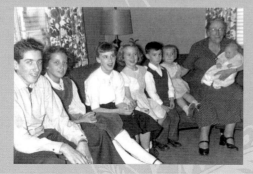

Janet at age 5 (fourth from left) with her two siblings and four cousins while visiting her paternal grandmother in October 1954.

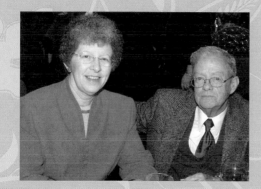

Janet and husband Chuck Bruner enjoyed a holiday celebration with colleagues from Neuro-Oncology and Neurosurgery in December 2001.

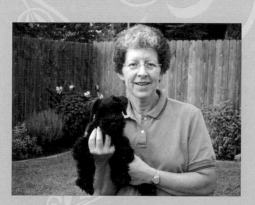

Janet holds Louis, a black miniature schnauzer, on his first day at home in June 2006. Louis' favorite activity is daily walks with his humans.

I am the oldest of three children, with a younger sister and younger brother. We grew up in a medium-sized Midwestern city in what I know now would be called a "middle class" neighborhood. Neither of my parents had the opportunity to attend college. My Dad certainly could have succeeded, but he graduated from high school at the depths of the Great Depression and chose instead to find a job and help put his younger sister through college. (She became a teacher.) Serving in World War II, my Dad was uprooted from his Midwestern life and stationed in Virginia, where he met my Mom. They married during the war and were separated for a time, of course. On returning home, my Dad resumed his job as a retail store manager, one he held for over 40 years, until he retired at age 65. My Mom also was a high school graduate. My parents' limited educational opportunities made them both determined that their children would not have the same limitations. It was always assumed that we would all go to college and even beyond. We were never forced — it was just a given. In our cases, the expectation worked. My sister has a Ph.D. and has been on the faculties at Harvard University and at the Massachusetts Eye and Ear Infirmary. My brother has an M.B.A.

I was a pretty quiet child and enjoyed reading. I especially loved Sherlock Holmes mysteries, and I think that love of mysteries contributed significantly to my life and my choice of a career. After all, pathology as a medical specialty involves continuously solving mysteries. Every case is an unknown, a puzzle to be solved.

I always preferred science to the humanities. To me, science was so much cleaner, neater and more logical. When it came time for me to choose a college and a major, my Dad in his practicality (especially since he had two other children to send to college) told me to choose some field that would allow me to go out and get a "good job" after graduation. I chose to major in pharmacy, as it seemed to fit both the "science" and "job" criteria. I attended the University of Toledo in my hometown and was a commuter student, as I didn't have the chance to live on campus. During my first year of college, I found a job with one of my early mentors, Dr. Gerald Schumacher, in a laboratory and had my introduction to research. I still remember doing a series of experiments to determine the concentration of a chemical in a solution using a spectrophotometer.

The summer after my first year of college, I had to find a job working in a pharmacy in order to start my internship. This internship had to be done over the summers following the first four years of the five-year pharmacy program. I found a great job in a small compounding pharmacy located in a medical building. At least I didn't have to also sell makeup and candy. All I had to do there was actually practice filling prescriptions. It was great! I worked at that same pharmacy during my entire college tenure. I also met my future husband, Charles Bruner, during that first summer, and we married soon after I graduated from college in 1972.

It was during my college years that I decided I wanted to do something other than just practice retail pharmacy as a career. I wanted to do scientific research and decided to pursue a Master of Pharmaceutical Sciences degree at the same pharmacy college where I had received my Bachelor of Science in Pharmacy. It was a new program, and I was the first student. I had a great experience and finished my degree, taking advanced courses and doing research, in two years. I thought about continuing study for a Ph.D. in pharmacy or a basic science, but after talking to several advisors and discussing the situation with Chuck, decided to attend medical school instead so that I would also have access to patients for clinical research. My plan was to do some sort of research in pharmacology, combining my pharmacy background with medicine and patient care. But life can change unexpectedly! As a second-year medical student at the Medical College of Ohio, I discovered pathology and, suddenly, I couldn't imagine doing anything else in medicine. I was fascinated to learn about the disease processes and how critical it is to have an accurate diagnosis as you begin treatment of the patient.

Everyone knows what a surgeon does and what a pediatrician does. But how many people — even medical students — really know what a *pathologist* does? I needed to find out, so I spent a year during medical school doing a pathology student fellowship. I had the wonderful opportunity of working alongside pathology residents, finding out what a pathologist's life is like and what they really do every day. I never looked back! Pathology has been my calling ever since. In addition to providing puzzles to solve, pathology is also a basic medical science with plenty of opportunities for scientific research.

I entered a pathology residency program and enjoyed learning both anatomic and clinical pathology. Initially I intended to specialize in forensic pathology, but I found the egregious brutality and bizarre trauma cases too difficult to endure on a daily basis. During those residency years, I met a young neuropathologist who encouraged me to think about neuropathology as a subspecialty. At the time, it seemed quite difficult and also quite esoteric, but gradually I began to appreciate the anatomic organization and functional intricacies of the brain and nervous system. I decided to enter a neuropathology fellowship. Up to that point, nearly my entire life had been spent in my hometown of Toledo, Ohio, but now I was forced to leave Toledo, as the city had no fellowships in neuropathology. I interviewed at several academic centers, but my choice of programs brought me to Houston and to Baylor College of Medicine. Baylor has an excellent and broad program in neuropathology, and so we moved from the North to the South, from cold weather to hot, from a small city to a massive one, and from cultural monotony to wondrous diversity.

During my two-year tenure at Baylor, I was one of three neuropathology fellows. We had two professors in the program (male and female), but the three of us spent the most time with Dr. Dawna Armstrong, and I think we all viewed her as our role model. She was (to us) the better diagnostician and was also quite serious about her research. She spent many didactic hours teaching us and preparing us to take our American Board of Pathology exams. It was during an elective period at Baylor that I came to M. D. Anderson Cancer Center for the first time and met Dr. Bruce Mackay, who at that time was chief of the Electron Microscopy section. He had an international reputation in the field, and I could not imagine being in Houston without learning from him. I was also nearing the end of my fellowship, and Dr. Mackay suggested that I might consider joining the Pathology department faculty at M. D. Anderson. He spoke to the chairman about this, and it seemed that there was a need for a neuropathologist to support a new effort in neuro-oncology and neurosurgery. I had always intended to return to Ohio to practice, but I couldn't pass up this opportunity at M. D. Anderson.

In my first few years at M. D. Anderson, I did general pathology diagnostics in addition to neuropathology, but the Brain Tumor Program eventually grew large enough to occupy all of my time. As the only neuropathologist here at that time, it was difficult for me to find others to help me as I continued to develop my diagnostic skills. However, I was fortunate to have many colleagues in the Texas Medical Center, and I was able to keep in close contact with my former mentors and associates. We formed a neuropathology group for the Houston-Galveston area, and we still meet monthly to exchange glass slides and discuss interesting or challenging cases.

I soon formed very rewarding collaborations with colleagues in the departments of Neuro-Oncology and Neurosurgery for research and for patient care. Several of us had laboratory programs, and we worked together to obtain a Program Project Grant for brain tumors that continued for about 10 years. We also initiated a tissue bank for human brain tumors that still exists today and is utilized for research efforts by the entire Brain Tumor Program. Both of these departments grew rapidly, and, as the only pathology support for their collaborative research, I was overwhelmed with riches. By the late 1980s there was too much work for one person. Fortunately, I was able to justify my need for help and recruited two additional neuropathologists in the early 1990s.

The late 1980s to mid-1990s was a significant period for my career development. I was an associate professor, and my research was going well, especially with collaborations in the Brain Tumor group. I was also asked to be an editor for a major textbook on neuropathology, a significant and rewarding effort. I owe much gratitude to the Pathology department chairman and division head at that time, Dr. John Batsakis, for some events that took place. He and I both happened to be "early birds" and were in the office by about 6 a.m. each day. He was in the habit of having coffee with several other senior faculty at around 7 a.m. in the cafeteria. Since my office happened to be next door to his, one day he stopped and asked me to join their informal group. Those informal discussions over coffee contributed significantly to my knowledge and growth in the areas of institutional issues and politics. I became acquainted with more faculty outside my department. Dr. Batsakis also made sure that I was invited to serve on institutional committees. Although I can't say that every minute spent on every committee meeting was entirely productive, I was able to meet lots of faculty and administrative folks from across the institution, and this has continued to be of great benefit to me in my career.

One day during another conversation with Dr. Batsakis, he gave me some advice on what I should do if I ever aspired to be a department chair in the future. I recall that my immediate response to him was that such an aim was definitely *not* in my career plan. However, I never forgot that conversation, and, within a year or so, I knew that this, in fact, *was* something I eventually wanted to do and needed to prepare myself for. There were few leadership courses at M. D. Anderson in those days, and few women were invited to attend the one that we developed with Rice University. There were certainly no pathologists invited to that course! I heard about the American College of Physician Executives and its excellent series of courses available at various locations across the United States. I began taking many of those courses and considered working toward an M.B.A. at that time. I learned much from such diverse offerings as "Managing Change and Innovation," "Communication Skills," and "Health Law." I continued taking courses for several years but never made the commitment to an advanced degree. I nevertheless believe that this experience benefited me the most in the role that I have now. It also taught me that you need to be persistent in finding what you think you need to move forward. You can't let roadblocks get in your way.

Another key event that proved to be beneficial for me arose from my frustration with the organization and with my job during this period. I decided to consider a major relocation, sought out opportunities for positions with more administrative responsibility, and interviewed for several. In doing this, however, I came to realize what a wealth of professional opportunities we have at M. D. Anderson that are not really available at other academic institutions. Nevertheless, I am glad that I looked outside, as this allowed me to make a more informed decision to remain here.

Another seminal event in my career was the retirement of Dr. Batsakis in 1996 and the decision by our administration to unite the divisions of Pathology and Laboratory Medicine into one. Because the search for a new division head was destined to be an extended one, there was a need for an *ad interim* department chair of Pathology. I wanted to try that position but wasn't given the opportunity. In retrospect, I am grateful for that turn of events, as I have since been advised that a temporary appointment is not always the best path to the permanent position. The department remained in a period of turmoil for two years. When the decision was made to actively search for a division head, I applied for that position, prepared myself for the interviews, seriously designed my strategic plan and vision for the division, and failed to get the job. Nevertheless, the process itself was of great value to me, and I am sure that those from our administration and the search committee who talked with me came to have a different, and more positive, view of me through that process. Because of those interviews and that extensive preparation, I was named the department chair of Pathology after the new division head had been hired. That was in late 1998, and I was the first woman faculty member to chair a clinical department.

I knew that I could not continue to do everything I had been doing and still successfully lead a large department that had significant problematic issues at that time. I decided not to give up my patient care duties, as I needed to know firsthand what problems the other pathologists faced in their daily work. I also couldn't sacrifice education, as the department had and still has a large clinical fellowship program, and we all teach these fellows. I decided that I would cut back on my independent research and move more toward collaborative efforts. I considered my most important job to be developing the careers of my faculty members.

My first few years as a department chair were difficult. We needed to recruit faculty. We made significant changes in our workflow and organization. We also made changes in our educational programs. Moreover, although I was a professor of pathology, most of the department faculty who were senior to me were men, but this turned out to be less of a problem than I had feared. Each faculty member is an expert in a subspecialty area of pathology, and I believe this enhances both our respect for each other and our collegiality within the department. In fact, the first significant change we made as a department was to subspecialize our clinical practice in pathology. This served to make our patient care more efficient and utilized our expertise more effectively. It also strengthened our individual ties to the patient care and clinical research programs. As the number of faculty grew rapidly over the first four years, I had to learn to effectively delegate to leaders in each of our sections of pathology. We had managed to recruit and designate some excellent mid-level and junior pathologists, and I have been delighted with their growth as professionals. I used my learned leadership skills to help some other faculty move into more significant leadership roles.

Over the succeeding five years, the Pathology department faculty has continued its rapid expansion. We have now nearly doubled the number of faculty that were here when I became the chair. The opening of the Mays Clinic has had a significant impact on us, since we now have large patient care operations there as well as at the Alkek Hospital. We have had to duplicate our services and spread ourselves thinner. The move toward more formal programmatic organization of research has also affected the department, as the research laboratories of the faculty are now spread throughout the campuses. This makes it difficult for patient care faculty to preserve time for laboratory research. We are trying to use digital media strategies to address some of these challenges, but we are also continuing to add faculty to allow everyone to have sufficient protected time for academic productivity.

Coping with such a large operation has forced me to continue my education in leadership and management. Fortunately, M. D. Anderson has also recognized the need for such programs, and now we have our own courses. I use my organization skills to increase my own efficiency and am a master of multitasking (I never attend a meeting without taking along a few articles to read in case the discussion becomes dull). I delegate as much as possible, try to choose the right people for assignments, and give them as much freedom as possible to succeed. However, I do have to make an effort to refrain from micromanaging — it's my worst tendency.

I maintain my balance by trying to accomplish as much as I can during the week while making every effort to reserve my weekend time for my husband and my dog. I love being outdoors, plants and gardening. I don't have much garden space, but I do have lots of houseplants. I also love animals, especially dogs. As a child, I never had a dog. We got our first miniature schnauzer when I was a medical student and have had one or two in the house ever since, for the past 34 years. They have been a great joy to me, and I've learned from them, too. I walk with my dog Louis every morning, and that wakes me up. I have trained them all in competitive obedience and have showed them in obedience trials. Training the dogs in obedience has taught me the power of positive reinforcement and consistency. I have found that these supportive techniques are equally effective with people — even faculty pathologists!

Perhaps because of the scope and importance of the mission we are involved in, developing a successful career at M. D. Anderson is a challenge for all faculty. There is always more work than we can do and always more fascinating research than we can support. Success requires careful selection, blending and balancing of all these factors. And, finally, we need to develop fruitful collegial relationships and make sure that we save time for personal growth as well as our academic careers.

Sharon Y. R. Dent, Ph.D.

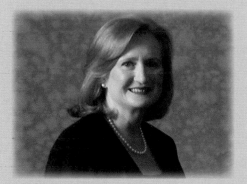

**Professor of Biochemistry and Molecular Biology
Rebecca Meyer Brown and Joseph Mellinger Brown
Chair in Basic Science Research**

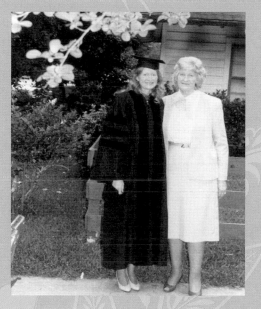

Receiving her Ph.D. from Rice University in 1986 was a wonderful day for Sharon and her proud mother, Rosie.

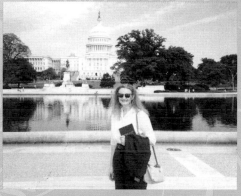

Sharon visited many historic sites in Washington, D.C., while completing a senior staff fellowship at the National Institutes of Health in nearby Bethesda, Maryland.

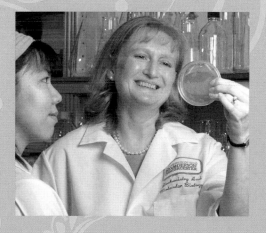

Mentoring graduate students in her laboratory has allowed Sharon to demonstrate her passion for research and teaching future scientists.

(Photo by F. Carter Smith)

knew from an early age that I would likely be an educator, although as a child growing up in Garland, Texas, I did not even know what a Ph.D. was. Education always equaled opportunity in my parents' eyes. As children of the Great Depression, Mom and Dad had to work hard to help keep food on the table, and neither was able to take their schooling as far as they might have wished. It is not surprising then that they taught their children that education is a gift, not an entitlement, and that we should take full advantage of any educational opportunities that came our way. They also tried to make learning fun. As a young girl back in the 1960s, I remember my dad using his new reel-to-reel tape recorder to help me record my voice as I read. I enjoyed hearing my words come out of the little electronic box; we must have spent hours doing that. My mom helped instill a love of reading by taking us to the library at least once a week once we were in school. In fact, if we were good and did all of our chores, instead of allowances we got to go to the library and check out *any book we wanted*. Books were real treats to us.

Looking back, I realize now that my parents also introduced me to science. Both Mom and Dad loved nature and would take us to the zoo, the aquarium, or the natural science museum in downtown Dallas every couple of years, so we came to look forward to this event and enjoyed it. My interest in science and math really blossomed in high school under the influence of three special teachers: Ms. Mathews (biology), Mr. Stockton (organic chemistry) and Mrs. Langston (algebra). On their blackboards, these potentially tedious subjects came alive, and I went off to college thinking that I would become a science teacher myself.

So how did I instead end up with a Ph.D. in biochemistry? Two closely related events changed my mind. First, I went to see my college career advisor to discuss the courses I needed to take to earn my degree in science education. I clearly remember walking into her office with a list of courses I had picked out and then watching in astonishment as she struck through all the science courses one by one and replaced them with education courses. I asked her how I would possibly be able to teach science if I did not study it myself, and she assured me that it was not necessary to understand science to be a science teacher. At that point, I began to think that perhaps I had chosen the wrong career path.

Shortly thereafter, I saw an advertisement for an open work-study position in a biochemistry lab on campus. I applied and was called in to interview with Myron (Mike) Jacobson, a young assistant professor. I was nervous, thinking that he would ask me a lot of questions about biochemistry. Instead, he gave me an even bigger scare — he asked me if I could type. (Since this was before the days of word processing, I hardly blame him for trying to find someone to help him prepare his grants, lectures and papers.)

However, typing was the only course I had ever dropped because of poor performance; in fact, I think I made history at my high school when I dropped out of typing and into trigonometry!

I confessed to Dr. Jacobson that I could not type, but he hired me anyway and turned me over to his technician, Rodney Barton, who showed me the laboratory and explained how things worked. Rodney then gave me my first assignment, a paper chromatogram. Rodney showed me how to spot the sample onto the paper with a capillary pipette and told me that it was very important to let the spot dry completely before applying the next aliquot. It was a fairly large sample, and the capillary pipette was very small, so it took me hours to spot the entire thing. But I loved every minute of it! It was the first time I had the chance to participate in a real experiment. In hindsight, I can't help but wonder if that first task had been a test of my dedication and patience. Little did they — or I — know that it would be a turning point in my life. I literally fell in love with science in that lab, and I knew then that it was my true calling. Who would have thought that not being able to type would lead to a scientific career?

Mike and his wife, Elaine (also a scientist and professor), were great mentors, and they encouraged me to apply to graduate programs. I decided to apply to the Ph.D. program at Rice University because of the school's outstanding reputation in biochemistry and in the sciences in general. I also needed to stay in Texas, and Rice was (and still is) one of the best universities in the state. I was very honored to be accepted. Although my parents were not sure what I would do with a Ph.D. in biochemistry and certainly did not like the idea of their middle child moving to Houston to live by herself (during my last semester at college, Dad actually started sending me newspaper clippings about shootings and other crimes in Houston), they supported my dreams. So we loaded up Dad's pick-up, and we headed south.

As a Ph.D. student at Rice, I found another great mentor, Dr. Susan Berget. Sue is well known for discovering RNA splicing during her postdoctoral studies with Phil Sharp at MIT. She had joined the faculty at Rice not long before I joined her lab. I learned a lot from Sue, not only in terms of science but also what it takes to set up a new lab, get your first paper published in the face of powerful competitors, and achieve tenure as a molecular biologist in a department focused primarily on classical enzyme kinetics.

I also met my first husband in Sue's lab. He was a senior undergraduate doing his honors thesis when I was coming in as a first-year Ph.D. student. We had many mutual friends and scientific interests, so we got to know each other over the next couple of years. A few years later, as we were completing our Ph.D.s, we got married. I received my degree, but my husband was in the M.D./Ph.D. program at Baylor College of Medicine, so we needed to stay in Houston a bit longer so he could complete his M.D.

I looked for a postdoctoral position close by. My plan was to complete a short postdoctoral training position in Houston and then do a second one if necessary before looking for a faculty position. Sue and some other members of the advisory committee at Rice were somewhat worried that I took this course of action. It was unusual at that time to do more than one postdoc, and doing so was often considered to be a sign of deficient ambition or scientific aptitude. However, I was intrigued by the science going on in the lab of a relatively new assistant professor at Baylor named David Allis, so I saw the situation as an "opportunity" to work with him. That decision turned out to be another major turning point in my career, as David became a lifelong mentor, friend and advocate.

It is hard to talk about David Allis without using superlatives. He is the very personification of enthusiasm. He is a fantastic scientist and an outstanding teacher. I thought I loved science when I joined his lab, but he showed me what real scientific passion is. Not only did he work very hard, but also he took real pleasure in every experiment and every new piece of data generated. (He still does.) He expected everyone in his lab to work hard, too, but he never asked anyone to do anything that he was not willing to do himself. I began my work in the area of chromatin in Dave's lab. At that time, his research was focused on histone modifications in a ciliated protozoan called *Tetrahymena thermophila*. My work with these little swimming creatures was vastly different from my work with HeLa cells in Sue's lab. Perhaps this lab was where I first recognized that each model system has value and that using more than one system opens up powerful research possibilities. My own work today uses mice, yeast and mammalian cell cultures. I firmly believe that the use of these multiple systems is necessary to get needed answers to important questions.

After my husband finished his M.D./Ph.D., we were faced with the challenge of finding two scientific positions in the same city. We chose to take fellowships at the NIH in Bethesda, Maryland. My parents were again worried, because I was moving away from Texas for the first time. In their minds at least, I was moving to the far North.

At the NIH, I worked with Robert (Bob) T. Simpson. Bob was unique: he allowed his fellows total freedom in their studies. He was always available if I wanted to talk, but he gave me free reign in my research. He supported my desire to learn about yeast genetics and even paid for my training in a three-week course at Cold Spring Harbor. My time in Bob's lab was the most fun I ever had doing research. The NIH had a strong and interactive community of chromatin researchers, and I had no responsibility other than to do what I wanted to do. I was part of Bob's group for five years, and from him I learned the value of letting people grow into themselves. Once again,

I had chosen a wonderful, talented and caring mentor.

After leaving the NIH, my husband and I again had to find two positions in the same city, this time at the assistant professor level. We talked about different strategies for our job search. Should we send in our applications together? Should we limit ourselves to specific cities with large medical centers that were likely to have jobs available for us both? Or should we just both go for the best jobs we could, and then sort out what the other person would do? We ended up doing the latter, and, to our surprise, multiple opportunities for dual positions presented themselves. In the end, it came down to a choice between two positions in the same department at the University of Michigan in Ann Arbor or two completely independent positions back in Houston. We both loved Ann Arbor, and the science there was quite strong. However, neither of us liked the idea of constantly being compared with one another within the same department as we worked towards tenure. Also, we both had aging parents back in Texas. And although we knew that we could handle the Texas heat, we were not so sure about the Michigan winters. So, for a combination of reasons, we headed south once more.

I started my lab at M. D. Anderson Cancer Center in 1993. If I had to use one word to describe my time here, it would be "opportunity." I have been able to expand my research program in ways I had never imagined when I first started. The institution has nurtured my career with pilot project funding and developmental awards and has celebrated my successes. I have had great students and fellows in my lab, and, through my participation in the UT Graduate School of Biomedical Sciences, I have at last achieved my original goal of becoming an educator.

I really enjoy several aspects of my career. First, of course, is the science. I love a good experiment and still get "jazzed" by discovery. Second, I love that I get to travel and meet other scientists from all over the world. Who would ever have thought that this Texas girl would one day travel to Beijing for a genetics conference and have the chance to stand on the Great Wall of China? Third, I get to work with bright and excited young scientists. Their enthusiasm continually inspires me.

Have I had disappointments? Certainly. Are there things I would do differently? Yes. In retrospect, I would have taken time to have children when I was young. My grandmother had eight kids and my mother had five. I thought I would be able to have children whenever I was ready, but I did not want to take time out for a baby when I was doing my graduate work or my postdoctoral training, so I put it off until my mid-30s, after I had taken my faculty position. It never occurred to me that I would run out of time. Before I knew it, I was 39, childless and "newly single." My biological clock was real, and it had run out.

Another thing that I would change if I could would be the lack of self-confidence that's followed me for most of my career. As a student, a postdoc, and an assistant professor, I was always worried about not knowing enough and making mistakes. It wasn't until my 40s that I gave myself permission to be human. Paradoxically, accepting my weaknesses has actually made me a stronger scientist, mentor and person.

Finally, I wish that earlier on I had spent more time just enjoying life. After my divorce, I decided to do something I had always wanted to do — take dancing lessons. Now I love to dance. I also met my new husband in dance class, and dancing is something we enjoy together. I also enjoy my dog and my hobbies, like quilting. Like my parents, I love nature and enjoy visiting natural wonders such as the Grand Canyon. I have vowed to take time to enjoy these things as I move through life, just as I enjoy my career.

As to my goal for the future, I am not a terribly sophisticated person, and fittingly, my motto is one that I saw on a frozen pizza box back when I was a student. We ate a lot of frozen and fast food in those days, and one brand of pizza we liked was Rose Totino's. Rose's motto was: "Be the best and be generous." That sounds like a good plan to me.

Carmen P. Escalante, M.D.

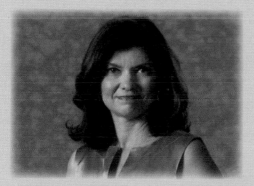

Professor and Chair of General Internal Medicine, Ambulatory Treatment and Emergency Care

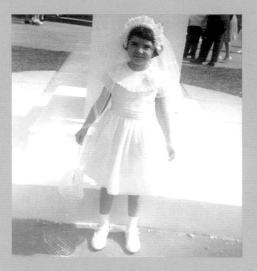

Carmen was 6 when she took her first communion in May 1966.

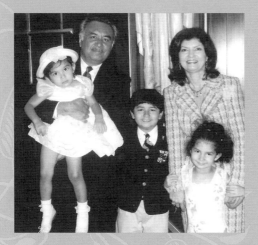

In May 2007, Carmen and husband Ramon celebrated the first communion of their son Damaso, shown with sisters Caroline (in Ramon's arms) and Isabella.

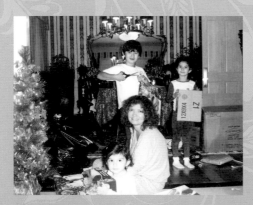

Opening gifts on Christmas Eve 2006 was another special time for Carmen and the three children.

As I reflect on my life and career, I silently chuckle at how unbelievable it all seems. I never planned for or dreamed of a career in academic medicine. I never thought that I was smart enough. I decided to go to medical school because I had always wanted to take care of patients. Although I do a lot less of it now than I did at the start of my career, caring for patients still gives me much satisfaction, and I believe that my work as an administrator and researcher still ultimately impacts patient care. That aspect is extremely important to me. The key to my success has been being able to identify and respond to the right opportunities.

I grew up in a small town in southern Louisiana, the oldest of six children. Neither of my parents attended college. My father received his high school equivalency while he was in the Navy, and my mother did not complete hers until I was in medical school. But my parents both valued education and made it clear to their children that we would attend college.

My mother was very influential during my childhood. I remember her continual encouragement to "do your best at whatever you do." (I frequently hear myself repeating those "mom phrases" to my own children — and it's rather scary to hear Mom's words echoing in my home.) My mother was a housewife, and her focus was on maintaining our home and rearing her children. She was always caring for us, and, as the oldest sibling, I often helped her look after my brothers and sisters. (I still remember changing their cloth diapers.) We were expected to help out around the house. My sisters and I took turns drying dishes, dusting furniture and ironing clothes, and my two brothers emptied the trash and mowed the lawn. But Mom did the bulk of the work — she saw us off to school every day and did the cooking, washing and cleaning. Housekeeping, though, never appealed to me. I decided early in life that I wanted something different. I was very shy, quiet and serious as a child. I was a straight-A student and became quite upset whenever I received a B. I still remember receiving a B in math for the first quarter of seventh grade. I was very unhappy and studied extra hard to have an A the remainder of the year. I still set high standards for myself and believe it was my mother's constant encouragement to strive for the best that instilled that drive in me.

One of my high school chemistry teachers was instrumental and a mentor in guiding me toward a medical career. I also had a high school math teacher who encouraged me. Both were women and had succeeded in education careers centered on science and math. I enjoyed chemistry and math and was very successful in these classes. I am sure some of my enjoyment was due to these two ladies and the mentorship they provided me. For me, this was when the light bulb went off. In junior high school, I decided that I wanted to be a doctor, and I never wavered from that goal afterward. I have no regrets about my decision and am thankful that these teachers saw my potential and helped me to see it, too. Very few students in my hometown attended medical school. I graduated from high school in 1977 as class valedictorian. Never the cheerleader, the prettiest, or the most vivacious, I was known as "the smart one" by my classmates.

All of my siblings and I attended college, and five of us received our degrees. I went to a local college, Nicholls State University in Thibodaux, Louisiana, on a full academic scholarship. I worked part time as a surgical clerk at the local hospital, which not only afforded me extra money to help defray expenses but also allowed me to develop some insights into what a medical career might really be like. Finances were always a concern, especially since our family was large and my father was not highly paid. However, we were always comfortable, happy and loved. I studied hard, lived at home and continued to save money so that I could pay for medical school. I met many new friends during my undergraduate days, and several of us were accepted into the same medical school class. Although I majored in chemistry and took numerous math courses, I also really enjoyed some of my fine arts electives, especially Latin. (Later in life, when I have more time for myself, I would like to explore the humanities and arts further. Recently, while helping my son study ancient Greece for his third grade class, I realized just how interesting his homework projects are to me.)

In 1981, I graduated from Nicholls State *summa cum laude* and then went on to Louisiana State University Medical School in New Orleans. It took me awhile to realize that my medical school classmates were a lot smarter than the students I had known in my college days. I studied hard and focused on my goal of graduating and becoming a doctor. This was also the first time I had lived away from home, and I quickly learned how to do my own laundry and cook my own meals. I also appreciated my parents a lot more after I left home.

After graduating from medical school in 1985, I moved to Houston to complete a residency in internal medicine at The University of Texas Health Science Center. I moved here along with two good friends from my medical school class, and we all went through the same internal medicine training. (One of these friends, Dr. Kristen Price, would later join me here at M. D. Anderson, where she is now a department chair.) Having good friends then was a great way to decompress and reflect on our lives and careers. We were busy, with lots of work and very little sleep, but we enjoyed and made the most of our small bits of free time.

Although I learned a lot about taking care of patients, I was happy when I finally completed my residency. I joined M. D. Anderson in 1988, when the section of General Internal Medicine was in its infancy. At that time, the section had only two faculty members; today, there are more than 30. I learned a lot about the importance of networking, organizational structure and lines of authority very quickly. I also learned the significance of being a good communicator, regardless of whether the communication was directly related to patient care or to other issues. I was hired to be full-time patient care, and for the first seven years of my career, I was on service 12 months a year. I was very naïve then and did not understand the concepts of tenure and promotion. No one explained to me how these things worked. I was told that I was needed to take care of patients and that if I did this, I would do very well in the institution. It was only after about seven years that I realized that with changes in the divisional leadership, I was not going to be promoted if I continued only to see patients, as I had initially been asked to do. At this point I began reengineering my career to meet the necessary requirements for promotion. Unfortunately, my supervisor and I had not planned a pathway. I have learned from my own experiences, and now, as a department chair, I have discussions with my section chiefs and faculty regarding the expectations and advanced planning for promotion of every faculty member.

A hidden opportunity came early in my career when I was asked to participate as a member of the Disaster Committee. This committee has since been renamed and melded into others, but its purpose was to prepare for internal and/or external disaster type situations. Little did I know that this committee appointment would mushroom to many others over my career. I chaired the committee for a few years and then went on to chair the Transfusion Committee, the Medical Practice Committee, the Credentialing Committee of the Medical Staff, and, currently, the Executive Committee of the Medical Staff. I really do believe my success in institutional and medical staff committee participation would never have happened if early on I had declined participation in the Disaster Committee. This was definitely an opportunity that I am glad I took advantage of years ago. Working on institutional committees involves a time commitment, but participating helped me to better understand the institution's organization and mission, network and form alliances with numerous colleagues, and develop my leadership skills. Chairing a committee of faculty is not an easy task — at times, it can be like herding cats. Listening to various viewpoints, keeping the focus on the issue at hand, and moving the agenda forward as the clock ticks are skills developed only with practice.

A major change in my career occurred in 1997, when I was given the opportunity to be the section chief of General Internal Medicine. At that time, we had perhaps five full-time physicians in the group. I had never managed anyone but accepted the challenge and learned on the job. It was a trying first year for various reasons, and I learned many things by trial and error. But I was a quick learner, and if I made a mistake, I did not repeat it.

Over the next few years our section began to grow, and a feeling of camaraderie developed. I sapped up as much knowledge as I could from anyone around who seemed to be successful. Learning by observation can be very powerful. I also learned the importance of listening, which was a difficult skill for me to master. Although it seems simple, becoming a good listener takes patience and skill. I am similar to Pooh Bear in that I am one of very little patience, although not a bear. As you can see, my analogies are based on the influence of my children. However, over the years I have become a much better listener and have learned much more from listening than from speaking.

In 2000, the Division of Internal Medicine was created, the previous sections became departments, and I became the ad interim chair of the Department of General Internal Medicine, Ambulatory Treatment and Emergency Care. I served in this role until 2005, when I was appointed the permanent department chair. During my tenure as ad interim chair, I participated in several leadership seminars, including the Faculty Leadership Academy, which gave me an opportunity to learn new skills and refine those that I had already attained. It gave me time to reflect on my personal management style and its effectiveness and also allowed comparison with others in the group sessions. I highly recommend seizing any educational opportunities for leadership growth that present themselves.

Currently, our department is composed of five sections that include some 100 faculty (including vacant positions and consultants) and nearly 60 staff. I have developed and implemented new programs that have been successful in integrating internists in various necessary functions throughout M. D. Anderson (for example, perioperative assessments, hospitalist program, and the Suspicion of Cancer Clinic), and I have recently realized that I really enjoy this administrative work. I am also working to build a stellar research component in our department to complement the top-notch clinical program we have already built. Hiring faculty with a similar vision, enthusiasm and motivation is essential and allows me to delegate tasks without having to worry about doing everything myself. Delegation takes some practice. Initially, it was difficult for me to hand projects over to others because I was used to doing everything myself, and I felt that I could do it better than anyone else. I also suspect that I was somewhat insecure in handing off something that was my responsibility. But once I started delegating certain tasks to very capable individuals, I soon learned how it benefited all of us: I had more time to focus on the things that really needed my full attention, and the people following my directions were able to grow in their own leadership capabilities by leading projects of their own.

I enjoy helping our faculty plan their career paths, whether for the short- or long-term. To be successful, young faculty must recognize that developing their interests and integrating these interests with the department's goals will lead to promotion and/or tenure. I have a significant number of faculty in my department who are women. I have always chosen the best candidate for a job, irrespective of gender; however, many of the best candidates have been women. Perhaps women are attracted to opportunities in settings where there are more successful and happy women, and so perhaps we have been able to grow our numbers due to this influence.

Reflecting on my career nearly 20 years after I first started as an instructor of medicine, I believe that things could have been easier. I really never had a specific mentor, a sage I could always turn to for advice. I have modeled myself after numerous people, and many of them probably never knew that they helped script my success. I am like a sponge, and I absorbed from others the good things that I thought were working.

In 1994, I married a wonderful man who has added balance to my life and has frequently been a great sounding board. He has also been exceptionally supportive of my career and has encouraged me to take on new challenges. An attorney with past banking experience, he founded a building company, so our two busy careers have continued in parallel.

Our first child, a son, was born in 1999. I had never appreciated all of the complexities of being a parent until I became one myself. For me, being a mother is a lot harder than being a physician, but I love it and have never regretted it. It took some time to learn how to balance being a doctor, wife and mother, but it is not an impossible task. The art of multitasking is essential to being successful. I took 10 weeks of leave for my first child and was a nervous wreck when I returned to work. I suppose I was not totally confident that a nanny would take care of my son as well as I could. With time, however, this fear has been put to rest. I had two more children, daughters born in 2001 and 2004, and took leave to spend time with each of them after they were born. I would definitely encourage taking some needed time away when children are born. It is a special time, often hectic with transitions. I have learned that work goes on regardless, but this family time is irretrievable and will be gobbled up if not rightly preserved. When I returned to work following each leave, I felt ready and somewhat refreshed despite those early morning feedings.

With the addition of each of our children, our lives became a little more complicated, but my husband and I became more relaxed as parents. In addition to hiring a full-time nanny/housekeeper, I initially had a part-time cleaning lady to help with major cleaning, especially when the children were very young and not yet in school. My husband and I juggle our careers and divide the childcare tasks between us. He often comes home from his office to help with baths and then goes back to finish up work once they are in bed. I have become more relaxed about things — sometimes everything is not in its perfect place, but that is O.K. It is a trade-off that is sometimes necessary to enjoy our family *and* have a successful career.

This year my children are all in school. The two older children go a full day, while my youngest daughter is in an early childhood program that lasts until lunchtime. My husband and I have learned how to delegate tasks and trust a little more, and my nanny picks up my youngest daughter from school. I take my children to school in the morning, and my husband picks up the older two, helps them get started on homework, and then goes back to his office. I am a planner at heart, and I carefully organize my day so that I can be home by 6 p.m. and my nanny can leave. Finding a good nanny/housekeeper is an essential survival skill and will make you feel so happy and carefree. I have learned that I will never be able to finish everything in a day and must prioritize those things that are most important. This not only applies to my work schedule but also to home activities. I know that I would not be as good a mother or as happy a person if I gave up my career to be at home.

Frequently, my husband will give me advice if I have a particularly difficult issue, but we try not to discuss work; we'd much rather spend our scarce time focusing on our children. Often, we end up talking about which of us will attend the next school function or soccer game or about how we will get the three of them to their various activities. As a two-career family, having a full-time chauffeur at our disposable would be an ultimate dream.

At this time in my life, my hobbies are my husband and children. They are my passion, and I find extreme pleasure in spending time with them. For example, when I return home each evening, my children run to the door to tell me about their school day. This is a wonderful way to recharge for the evening. When the children are older and need less of my attention, I may refocus my hobbies, but for now there is no time and I readily accept this. I have two full-time jobs: my career as a physician and my job as a mom and wife. Both are non-stop, and both are exceptionally challenging, but both are also very satisfying.

I am very pleased with the path my career has taken. I enjoy my job and look forward to work every day. I never anticipated that my career would take this turn, but I am quite delighted with the results.

Varsha V. Gandhi, Ph.D.

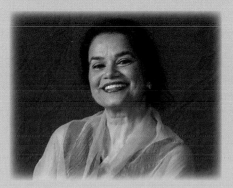

Professor of Experimental Therapeutics
Ashbel Smith Professor

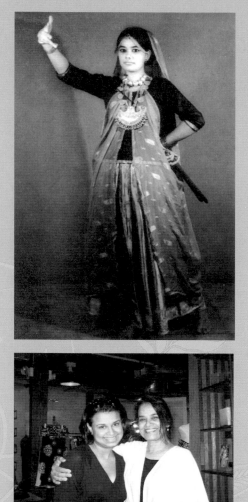

While growing up in India, Varsha was photographed holding two wooden sticks (Dandiya) in her left hand as she prepared to lead the group dance Dandiya Ras.

Varsha frequently visits New York City to spend time with daughter Meghana, who always has a new restaurant for them to try.

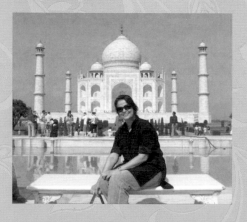

One of Varsha's favorite sites is the beautiful Taj Mahal, where she often takes M. D. Anderson colleagues when they attend conferences in India.

ad I been asked long ago whether I someday planned to become a faculty member at one of the world's premier cancer centers and, in addition, whether I planned to write a vignette of my life experiences, my answer would have been a screaming no! During my high school and early college years, I knew a little bit about research and cancer but nothing about M. D. Anderson Cancer Center. Today, I find myself in a profession that I savor every day, and this is the direct result of a combination of circumstances, opportunities and developing new interests.

Just before my birth, my parents moved from the Indian state of *Gujarat* to Delhi, the capital of India. Born at home with the help of a midwife, I was the second child and daughter of my parents. A few years later, my brother was born, and my parents were very happy that they now had a son who would carry on the work of their *Ayurvedic* medicine store as well as the family name. In the Indian culture, boys are considered more important than girls are. I am very proud of my parents for rejecting the age-old tradition of keeping girls uneducated and unchallenged and instead providing their two daughters with access to a great education.

Before I could start school, my parents moved from Delhi to Kanpur, a city in India's northeastern state of *Uttar Pradesh* (UP), the state that includes the world-famous Taj Mahal. So that I would not forget my mother tongue, my parents enrolled me in a school in which courses were taught in *Gujarati*. As there were no age requirements for admission into this small school, I started first grade at age four. My parents soon realized, however, that in order to assimilate with the people of the region, I needed to be fluent in the *Hindi* language, so they transferred me to an all-girls school where everyone spoke and learned in *Hindi*. I tried to make new friends, but the language barrier prevented many girls from asking me to join their already-established groups. Resolute, I forced myself to rapidly learn the language. In this way, my early school years taught me to overcome obstacles with determination and to assimilate and enjoy a new culture. Many years later, I found these lessons useful when settling in America.

After high school, I wanted to go straight to medical school, but I was too young to enroll. After earning a bachelor of science degree in two years, I again considered this. Disappointingly, though, I discovered that in addition to the money needed for tuition, books and supplies, my parents had to first donate a huge sum of money to the medical college before I could be accepted. Student loan programs did not exist in India, and I was aware of my parents' financial situation, so I dropped the idea of becoming a physician. Instead, I enrolled in a two-year program leading to a master of science degree at Christ Church College, one of the top-ranked colleges affiliated with Kanpur University. Inspired by the teachers in the undergraduate classes, I chose a concentration in botany. At one point, I considered teaching that subject for the rest of my life after completing my graduate degree.

The results of my master of science degree examinations were fantastic. Not only had I earned first division (top-tier) honors in my degree program, but also I was ranked first among all botany master's students at Kanpur University. My friends and family were proud of my accomplishments, and I was relieved, as I had disappointed both myself and others by not receiving first division honors previously, including in my undergraduate work. Celebrations of my achievements were short-lived, though, as I applied for but did not receive a teaching job in the botany department of a local college. Many of my classmates had also applied for this position, but as it turned out, the successful applicant knew a city leader and had him push her application. This was my rude awakening to the fact that having outstanding credentials, though necessary, is not always sufficient to land a job.

Since I was without work, I decided to continue my graduate studies. Delhi University, one of the best universities in India, accepted me into its botany doctoral program with a scholarship. I was assigned a supervisor as well as a Ph.D. project on which to work. Life in Delhi brought excitement in the form of new experiences, both educational and social. My recently constructed hostel (dormitory) housed an amalgam of individuals from all over the world; now, English — not *Hindi* — was the main language of communication on campus. The botany department took up an entire building, not just a single floor, and my research project involved the challenging and interesting work of both histo- and biochemistry. Though great in these respects, Delhi University had no air-conditioned buildings, and there was no running water in my third-floor lab. On scorching summer afternoons, temperatures in the upstairs laboratories were sometimes higher than temperatures outside, reaching up to 46°C (115°F). Moreover, some of my histochemistry procedures required washing glass slides in running water five to six times; each time, I had to walk downstairs to the ground floor and then climb all the way back up. Such adverse conditions implanted "work-hard" genes in me; such traits are a must for success in any career and particularly for research, which demands a high level of energy, as it is constantly changing.

While still finishing my thesis, I received a job offer to be a lecturer (assistant professor) at *Daulat Ram College*, an all-girls college. Even though it was an *ad hoc* position, I took the job because I knew that once my thesis and viva examination were finished, I would be considered a prime candidate for a full-time position. (A viva is a final oral examination conducted by a faculty member from outside the candidate's university.) Although I enjoyed things like being around students (to whom I became a role model and mentor), teaching my favorite subject, and wearing beautiful *saris* and matching jewelry, I knew that someday I would tire of all this, since there was no creativity in what I was doing. I soon decided to abandon the monotony in favor of something that would never get old: research.

Toward the end of my doctoral studies, my uncle, who lived in Delhi, introduced me to his friend's son, who was visiting from America after completing his studies there and who subsequently became my husband. Ours was an arranged marriage, although not in the way often envisioned by Westerners. A couple of generations ago, it was true that parents arranged their children's marriages without the children's knowledge or consent. However, times have changed; in our case, we met several times, met each other's families, and independently decided to get married. The marriage brought me to America.

To a woman in her mid-20s arriving from a developing nation, the United States seemed the embodiment of luxury, opportunities and progress. I thought that there would be no barriers or boundaries to achieving success, but as I started to apply for jobs, I quickly realized that I had been idealistic. When I moved to Houston, I still did not have my Ph.D., as I needed to take a viva examination. Therefore, I was mostly applying for research intern or research assistant positions. Human resources staff at various universities told me that I was overqualified, did not have enough relevant experience, and/or lacked the necessary communication skills. Changing my tack, I decided to reach out directly to faculty members. While I felt certain that they would notice the aforementioned deficiencies in my credentials, they would also see a researcher who was passionate about science, driven and determined to succeed, and prepared to start working immediately. This strategy worked, as I made several contacts with plant science faculty members and received a paid research internship that involved plant tissue cultures for biomass production at the University of Houston. While working, I audited biochemistry, molecular biology and other courses to gain a better understanding of the developments in these subjects in the United States. I realized that there were limited options for plant scientists in Houston, so I began to search for a postdoctoral position in molecular biology, once again by contacting faculty. When the opportunity arose, I became a postdoctoral fellow in molecular biology at Rice University, where I used Drosophila as an experimental model system. During this period, I achieved two milestones: first, I took and passed the viva and final examination for my Ph.D., which took place at the University of South Carolina. Second, during my time at Rice, I used the open spaces of the campus to learn how to drive.

Although the work and training at the University of Houston and Rice were good, my science did not have any direct applicability to human life, and I was not getting any quality mentorship. Moreover, being around the Texas Medical Center rekindled my desire to be in the medical field. I knew, however, that it would not be easy for a trained plant biochemist with some experience in Drosophila molecular biology to land a postdoctoral position in cancer research. Because my husband and I had a steady income from his job, he encouraged me to take a risk and look for work that I liked, even if it meant being unsalaried in the beginning. I landed a postdoctoral position as a volunteer in the laboratory of the late Dr. Grady Saunders, head of the Department of Biochemistry at M. D. Anderson Cancer Center. I worked on Wilms' tumor (a pediatric kidney tumor also known as nephroblastoma), and a few months later, Grady mentioned that he had included my name in a grant application. If it received funding, I would become a paid postdoctoral fellow in his lab. I felt confident that he would get the grant.

While waiting for Grady's grant to come through and before starting a family, my husband and I decided to visit Europe. We brought home more than 12 books from the public library and prepared for our journey. For five weeks, we traveled across Europe by Eurail, staying in unusual but inexpensive places and visiting many of the recommended sights. I knew that I loved new customs and cultures from when I was transitioning between Kanpur and Delhi and establishing myself in America, but until I visited Europe, I did not realize how much I enjoyed traveling and hopping from one country to another, admiring in turn each area's art, architecture and ambiance.

Upon returning to the United States, I discovered that Grady's grant had not been funded — yet another circumstance that affected the unfolding of my career. When Grady's wife, Dr. Priscilla Saunders, told him that her officemate, Dr. William (Bill) Plunkett, was seeking a postdoctoral fellow to work on cancer therapeutics, Grady mentioned that if I were interested in chemotherapy research, I should talk to Bill. The chance to work in the medical field excited me, and, without thinking or making an appointment, I walked into Bill's office, the fingers of my left hand crossed while those of my right held my résumé. I have never met a faculty member more enthusiastic about his or her research than Bill. In addition, as a third-year associate professor at that time, Bill was senior enough to mentor a new postdoctoral fellow and junior enough to have the time to do so. The field of research was patient oriented — fulfilling a passion I had always had — and I was thrilled to become a postdoctoral fellow in his group.

After a lag period spent learning about this new area of research, I entered a long phase of productivity in the field of experimental therapeutics. We worked on nucleoside analogues such as cytarabine, fludarabine, gemcitabine and cladribine; it sounds like "bine"-counting, but, in reality, I was counting my blessings. Our overall goal was to understand the metabolic and mechanistic aspects of each analogue in order to use the analogues optimally and effectively in the clinic as single agents or in combination with other chemotherapeutic agents. For example, based on the metabolic properties of cytarabine, I hypothesized that fludarabine would modulate the accumulation of cytarabine triphosphate. The fludarabine-cytarabine combination was tested in cell lines and then in primary leukemia cells; finally, we worked with our colleagues in the Leukemia department to design a protocol to move the combination regimen into the clinic. This clinical pharmacokinetics and pharmacodynamics work was published in the *Journal of Clinical Oncology*, and I celebrated the paper as my triumph, not because it was published in a journal with a high impact factor but rather because it was published in a journal that would have a great impact on clinical researchers and on patients. The combination was used as front-line therapy, further improved at M. D. Anderson, and tested in many cancer centers around the world. For the first time in my life, my research directly affected patients, which I found to be an extremely rewarding experience. The proverbial term for such investigations is translational research, and since then, this type of research has been the nucleus of my scientific endeavors.

In the midst of writing grants, designing protocols, writing manuscripts and traveling to present my work, a very precious thing happened in my life: I became the mother of a daughter, Meghana. It was difficult to balance family *and* work, although I loved both. At home, my husband helped me raise our daughter and do the chores. I wanted to spend as much time as possible with her before she grew up, so I sometimes took her with me on my trips, both domestic and international. While I worked during these trips, she either spent time with a babysitter, sat in the last rows of auditoriums to listen to my seminars, or — when she became old enough — visited places on her own. My colleagues, internal and external collaborators, and professional friends know her. I have many memorable pictures of her: with the late Nobel Laureate Dr. Trudy Elion (whose drug we were testing); with Dr. Emil J Freireich, dancing at an ASCO reception; with Dr. Michael Keating, rowing on a lake in Hamburg; with Dr. Steve Rosen — with whom I have been collaborating for a decade — on Hawaii's Big Island; with Dr. Bill Beck, who once arranged a stretch limo for us (mostly for her) to go to O'Hare Airport after my seminar at the University of Illinois in Chicago; and with everyone in Dr. Plunkett's and my labs. Today, she is a young woman, and we are the best of friends.

As my career progressed, I received valuable help from leading faculty in obtaining tenure and in acquiring an independent laboratory space. I held an assistant professor appointment for six years, an NTRA (non-tenured research appointment) for three years, followed by a tenure-track appointment for the next three years. At the end of the sixth year, Dr.

Robert Bast, who was then head of the Division of Medicine and ad interim department chairman, recommended that I be promoted to tenure-track associate professor. As required, he also appointed three faculty members to evaluate my credentials, and they unanimously recommended that I be promoted to associate professor with tenure. A tenured position at any university puts an individual within an elite group of faculty members, but at M. D. Anderson, tenure also meant that the institution would pay the salary of this faculty member.

Hence, a state educational and general (E&G) slot was mandatory for a tenured position; however, Dr. Bast informed me that he did not have a slot for me. This meant that I would have to pay 100 percent of my salary from grants, as I had been doing for the past six years as an assistant professor. I spent the next eight months educating myself about the mystery of E&G slots, writing numerous memos to Dr. Andy von Eschenbach (Executive Vice President and Chief Academic Officer), Dr. Margaret Kripke (Vice President for Academic Programs) and Dr. Fred Becker (Vice President for Research), and meeting with Drs. von Eschenbach and Bast. I learned that among 128 tenure-track assistant professors, I was one of only three who were paying their entire salaries from grant funds. Frustrated to see such disparities, I sent my curriculum vitae to senior faculty members such as Drs. Walter Hittelman, Waun Ki Hong, Marvin Meistrich, Ray Meyn, Raphael Pollock and Grady Saunders to get their opinions. The more I received confirmation of the strength of my case, the more I discussed the promotion with Dr. Bast. On January 30, 1998, he called to say that they had found a slot, and in September of that year, I received the coveted tenured position. The process had been a nightmare, but the outcome was a dream!

Until I joined a newly formed space committee, I did not know about the inequalities that existed in the distribution of laboratory space, a vital resource for scientists. When committee chairman Dr. Bill Klein learned that I did not have any assigned independent laboratory space, he encouraged me to obtain some, and together we formulated a plan for doing so. I gathered and presented information to Dr. Reuben Lotan, the deputy head of research for the Division of Cancer Medicine, who in turn discussed the idea with Dr. Kripke. I received laboratory space with the valuable help of these individuals.

Overall, it was not easy for me to procure resources or to progress in the cancer center's hierarchy for two main reasons. First, I continued to work in the same organization where I had been trained, and, second, my department lacked a permanent chairperson who could have advocated my case. Perhaps it would have been easier if I had moved to a new institution, at which point I would have received, upfront, a tenured position and laboratory space. My experience suggests that junior faculty interested in being promoted and in obtaining additional resources ought to look beyond their current organizations for opportunities.

All of these experiences have formed a foundation upon which I continue to build my career. Perhaps the narratives of my progress in life and work can be of some use to scientists who are at various stages of their careers — whether discovering the competitive field of cancer research, establishing themselves in their careers, or serving as advisors and role models to up-and-coming scientists.

I came from a city that had one public library (which was open only two or three days a week), electrical power shortages during the summer, and limited hours of running water each day. As a result, I never took for granted the incredible resources available in the United States. For me, it was — literally and figuratively — a rags-to-riches transition. I have been to many countries, and what the United States has to offer to a hungry and curious mind surpasses what is available in any other place. My education and training have benefited enormously from this country's wealth, and I see no reason why scientists who come to this country from other nations cannot make the most of state-of-the-art facilities and training opportunities.

I would also encourage foreign scientists, especially women, to network with colleagues who are knowledgeable about working in America. Not only are these colleagues cognizant of the operating procedures and the rules of the game at every step in an academic career — grant and manuscript writing, promotions, serving on committees, and vying for awards and honors, to name a few — but also they can act as conduits for these steps. I would not be where I am today without the superb support of Drs. Waun Ki Hong, Hagop Kantarjian, Michael Keating, Bill Klein, Margaret Kripke, Reuben Lotan, Bill Plunkett, Garth Powis, Steve Rosen and Liz Travis.

To junior faculty, the cancer research road may appear winding, difficult and scary. Successful scientists have all experienced the frustrations and sorrows of rejected manuscripts, unfunded grants and incorrect hypotheses. Do not let these discourage you, as cancer research is creative, enjoyable and rewarding. At this early professional phase, find the cancer field that fascinates you, and pursue projects that become your passion. It does not matter what you select; what matters is how passionate you are about your chosen field. Become industrious and productive in your research area, and strive to publish papers and obtain grant funding. Publications and grants will substantially enhance your curriculum vita, and in terms of career advancement, nothing can substitute for an outstanding CV. It acts as an advocate, a campaigner and a recommendation letter. Finally, select your mentors wisely, and remain connected with them — and I will underscore that I used the plural, not singular, form of the word. Yes, you will need more than one mentor to assist, guide, motivate and push you.

Collaborating with other scientists is critical in cancer research and easily feasible for mid-career scientists. Cancer is complex, and cancer research calls for multidisciplinary efforts. As we grow more focused on our research areas, we become specialists in particular fields; at the same time, our overall base of scientific knowledge narrows. With the amount of literature germane to each area of cancer research, it is almost impossible to keep up with your own field, let alone learn about others. Institutions ought to recognize the importance of collaborative, collegial and collective efforts, allowing mid-career scientists with varying specialties to combine their expertise and resources.

To senior faculty members — especially women, who have the inherent capability to care and give — let your research goals encompass teaching and mentoring. I serve as the director of education and faculty development for the Department of Experimental Therapeutics, and I feel that it is of paramount importance to inspire and educate students and trainees who will carry on our mission of making cancer history: combating and hopefully curing cancer. This is a monumental task, and therefore, we must ensure that the next generation of interested, inquisitive and intelligent researchers is ready to roll.

If you have read this chapter to its finale, you now know how my circumstances and interests have shaped my academic career. I have been incredibly lucky to have such a great professional life. It is doing what I love and loving what I do; it involves encountering challenges that make each project unique and surprises that make each day interesting; it has been full of motivating mentors and great lab team members; and, perhaps most important, it consists of translational research, which impacts the lives of patients.

Every morning I enter M. D. Anderson through the Clark Clinic lobby. I see patients sitting and waiting with their loved ones. Their eyes are filled with the hope that they have arrived at the best possible place for their cancers to be conquered. But soon enough many realize that cancer is cruel and that even the best cancer center may not be good enough to cure their disease. This is what drives me to work harder and more efficiently every day — both alongside and with my lab team members and my wonderful colleagues — to find new remedies, new regimens and new drug combinations for their diseases. Even the best cancer center has to become better to conquer cancer.

Elizabeth A. Grimm, Ph.D.

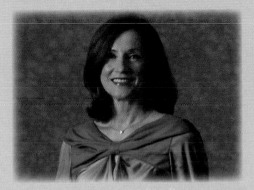

Professor of Experimental Therapeutics
Francis King Black Memorial Professorship
for Cancer Research

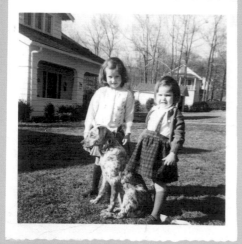

Elizabeth, left, and sister Susannah played with Freckles in front of the family home in Charleston, West Virginia.

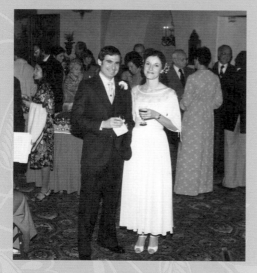

Elizabeth married Jack Roth, M.D., on Nov. 25, 1978, in Santa Barbara, California.

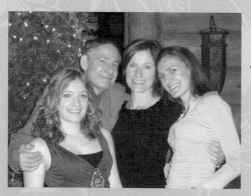

Jack, Elizabeth and daughters Katherine, left, and Johanna welcomed a new year (2006) in Telluride, Colorado.

Reflecting on my journey into cancer research, I am struck by how much serendipity, always planning for the future, an impatience for results, and a love of learning have served me well. I wish to share a glimpse of how, in my view, I have been able to achieve beyond my dreams to find success in "everything," which in the vernacular of my era meant a professional position, a husband and children. First and foremost, I enjoy scientific inquiry and love addressing molecular details. I was fortunate to learn critical hypothesis testing, which remains a key to public success. However, in the field of cancer research, the process is frustratingly slow, so I also take occasional risks by testing big leaps; this usually does not yield useful results, but it does provide some thrill of science. I also enjoy my fellow scientists, with whom I share my days, and thus, most of the time I feel that what I do is a pleasure (grant writing excluded) and a privilege rather than work.

I was born and raised in Charleston, West Virginia, where my father was an attorney and my mother was an English teacher. My mother taught school immediately after she graduated from college until my older brother was born, and then she stayed home and was busy with volunteer work and child care until my younger sister started junior high. When Mom returned to teaching, she quickly advanced to become the head of the English department at the city high school and also finished her master's degree. Even though many people perceived and still view the state of West Virginia as the illiterate center of the United States, my parents both had graduate degrees, and my siblings and I all knew that we were expected to attend both college and graduate school, which we did. Nevertheless, the field I eventually chose to pursue was new, and my parents questioned whether my Ph.D. in microbiology and immunology might prepare me to work at our local hometown hospital. They were understandably uninformed and uncomfortable as to how a cancer research career might proceed.

As a young child, I was either with my mother, who was usually reading, cooking and knitting, or with babysitters when Mom went about her volunteer and church activities. At an early age, I became my father's helper in the garden, as Mom was busy with Susannah, who was two years younger. Gardening was a hobby for both parents, as was playing the piano. Dad built a rock garden and a rose garden, tended beds of azaleas, and planted specimen trees. Mom tended flowering annuals and a few kitchen plants (rhubarb, green beans, tomatoes, mint, etc.), and particularly liked pansies. I greatly enjoy nature and outdoor activity, including gardening, and think there must be a "farmer" gene somewhere in me. Although both my parents had "achieved" in music activities in their youth, my Dad exhibited an innate ability not only to read music and play numerous instruments but also to "play by ear." One idea of childhood fun was for Dad to entertain the family with a series of medleys of popular music, often just heard that evening on the Ed Sullivan or Lawrence Welk shows. My sister and I would attempt to "sing and dance" on our stair landing as a stage — fortunately, home video equipment was not yet available! I think Dad was happy as an attorney, but I saw him and Mom both relaxed and happiest around the piano. I mention this since enjoyment of music remains a large part of my life, and I consider music one of the greatest cathartics. My childhood was filled with tennis, swimming, dogs, horses, music and many relatives. Although growing up in West Virginia could be considered a challenge from many perspectives, I was blessed to have a happy and stable family that provided me with resources to deal with life's later stresses.

My interest in science made me the "black sheep" of the family, as my sister (a psychology Ed.D.) calls me, since she and my older brother are both talented in the humanities. I believe that I was always curious about science and suspect that this was innate, as my environment was not structured to stimulate scientific inquiry. I do recall a personal curiosity and energy that led me to engage in early experiments. At the age of three, I escaped from my obligatory afternoon nap to perform a most memorable experiment, which almost set our house on fire. I was "testing whether paper would burn" by sticking a small piece into the pilot of a gas heater in our bathroom. Immediately realizing that paper did indeed burn, I threw it into the adjacent trash can, where it proceeded to set the contents on fire. My mother somehow became aware of this and quickly doused the burning trash can and overhanging curtains with buckets of water from the adjacent bathtub, saving the house and my still-sleeping baby sister. Ironically, my older brother and father were visiting the local fire station as part of a Boy Scout field trip and saw the alarm come in. They arrived at the house with the fire trucks just as Mom had totally extinguished the flames. Mom was the hero, and I was the culprit! Even today, my siblings tease me about this and are still jokingly reluctant to let me light the candles on birthday cakes.

My first trip outside West Virginia occurred when I was 13 and traveled by car with relatives to Myrtle Beach, South Carolina. The automobiles lacked air conditioning, and so six of us traveled with the windows down the entire way. I recall that the trip took a very long time, even necessitating a car repair on the way, so that our entire journey was over 20 hours. My Uncle Elmo did all the driving and must have been very tired. I also remember that our meals were picnics, packed by my mother and my Aunt Sarah, and that we ate lunch on a real picnic table by a stream while the car was being repaired. There was neither consideration to go to a restaurant nor to stop at a hotel or motel during the drive. When we arrived at Myrtle Beach in the middle of the night, I was totally awed by that first encounter with the ocean and have loved it ever since. My first experience living away from

Charleston, other than in the college dorm, was during the summer after my sophomore year in college; that summer I worked in Ocean City, Maryland, as a waitress at the original Phillip's Crab House. My mother and several of her friends came to "visit." Mom seemed to show up every time I had not been home for a few weeks. At the time, I did not read any meaning into her visits other than that she wanted to share in whatever I was doing.

The experiences of growing up in the small and comfortable environment of Charleston came to feel confining by my teenage years and led to my desire to become independent and look for travel, adventure and challenge. I now realize that in contrast to many others, I actively seek the challenge of change rather than being comforted by predictability. Although I am definitely not a thrill seeker by any means, I am rather easily bored and prefer to seek entertainment through active participation or thoughtful activities rather than passive ones.

Beginning with my generation, young women wanted even more than their mothers had experienced, especially the women at Randolph-Macon Woman's College (named change to Randolph College in 2007), from which I graduated in 1971. We were determined to plan for "everything" life had to offer. I am not sure whether it was the women's college environment, the liberal attitude of the early '70s, or sheer naiveté, but my classmates and I sincerely thought we could do anything and everything. One of the phrases popular at the time that (thankfully) I do not hear anymore was that now women could "bring home the bacon and fry it, too." I do think that, especially for my generation, the women's college environment was influential in that it provided us with female role models without the distraction of male competitors at that critical time of maturation. I obtained my degree in chemistry with a minor in music based totally on my interests and with no clear career path. Upon my parents' request that I consider a career as a high school chemistry teacher, I left college a semester early (having fulfilled all chemistry major and music minor graduation requirements) and enrolled in Marshall College (now Marshall University) to take teaching courses not offered at that time at Randolph-Macon, which was strictly liberal arts. I spent a semester "student teaching" and acquired a high school teacher's certificate in chemistry and physics, which was never officially used.

In college, I was attracted to a young man from a nearby university, and, immediately after my graduation in May, we were married (although the union was short lived) and I moved to Boston, where he was in medical school. It was this situation that led me, unexpectedly, to work in one of the best immunology research laboratories at Harvard Medical School; the lab was run by K. Frank Austen. A young female assistant professor in Dermatology, Irma Gigli, hired me as a technician, and this experience "set the stage" for my future. In my first year of working as a technician, I realized that my undergraduate education had been outstanding and on par with the "Ivy League" standards of those around me; when graduate student coworkers in that same lab encouraged me to consider applying to a Ph.D. program myself, my career direction and goal were finally defined. Meanwhile, the stresses of medical school and residency, along with mutual immaturity and my growing desire to apply to graduate school all contributed to the dissolution of my ill-fated marriage. We were both growing intellectually and emotionally, and I now believe that 21 is really too young for individuals to know themselves. My then-husband became uncertain of what his role would be were I to pursue an advanced degree. At one point, he asked, "Would I have to go to professional meetings with you?", suggesting that he questioned his status and that I might not be the doting spouse of his parents' generation. I now realize that this was also a difficult time for young men, as their traditional roles were being altered as well. At Harvard I was profoundly inspired by the realization that I was part of the vanguard of the application of molecular biology to the study of human disease and witnessed the very first attempts at isoelectric focusing as well as other early types of molecular studies.

In 1973, we moved to Los Angeles, where I was fortunate to work another two years while applying to the Ph.D. program of the UCLA Medical School (and finalizing my divorce). I worked in the laboratories headed by Donald Morton, chairman of the UCLA Surgery department at that time, and his junior faculty as they established immunotherapy and melanoma research programs. Although I left the study of melanoma and human cancer research during my Ph.D. dissertation years for transplantation immunology research, I have now returned to a singular melanoma focus and am extremely fortunate that Don Morton remains a world class leader in this area. I continue to apply much that I learned from his group then and now. As a full-time Ph.D. student then, I was most fortunate to have been accepted to do my dissertation research in the laboratory of Benjamin Bonavida, who was then a beginning assistant professor and now continues to be active as a professor at UCLA and is recognized as a world-class tumor immunologist. "Ben" remains a wonderful mentor and role model, not only for science itself, but also especially for his personal caring for students and teaching. I received encouraging awards, such as the UCLA "Graduate Woman of the Year" award, for publishing more papers than any other female Ph.D. candidate.

It was during these years in the lab at UCLA that I also met my wonderful husband, Jack Roth, who had left Johns Hopkins (where he had graduated with his M.D. degree and started his surgical residency) for a junior research fellowship, coincidentally in the same laboratory where I was then working.

Curiously, after we started dating some time later, he decided to stay at UCLA as a surgical resident. Jack shares my love of science and research, and since he was an only child whose Mom had worked full time, he had no problem with my pursuing a career and in fact was quite encouraging — then and now. We were married Thanksgiving weekend in 1978, in nearby Santa Barbara, California, which was as far as we could possibly go and still be back to work on Monday morning. Jack also shares my love of music, and, although we had only 30 guests at our wedding, we splurged on hiring a classical string quartet to play for the ceremony and another live band and vocalist for our dinner and dancing. The next spring, I finished my postdoctoral fellowship at the UCLA Molecular Biology Institute and began my first professional position, at the National Institutes of Health, in 1979. I assumed that I was going to do a second postdoctoral fellowship but quickly learned that I had been hired by Steve Rosenberg as the youngest member of "Cancer Experts" at the National Cancer Institute in Bethesda.

In Bethesda, Jack and I bought our first house and settled into happy years of building our careers, with dinners often at the health club after work and exercise, and season tickets to the National Symphony with the ritual drive down Wisconsin Avenue to the Kennedy Center. In 1982, when I was confident that I had a solid career, we began to consider that our lives might be enhanced by children, and in January 1983, our first daughter, Johanna, was born. I was totally naive about children and did not anticipate how much pleasure she (and later Katherine) would bring to us and our marriage. Jack and I were very fortunate to organize and afford a combination of domestic help, parents, in-laws, and advice from my sister to negotiate the early years of successful baby and toddler care. These were happy and active years during which I was very productive at work, having produced a series of *Journal of Experimental Medicine* papers that were recognized as "Citation Classics." Our second daughter, Katherine, was born in 1986, during our last months at the NIH, and when she was three weeks old, Jack and I brought her on the plane to Houston for a house hunting trip, as I was still nursing. Jack and I both had been recruited to M. D. Anderson Cancer Center during the previous year, and we finally decided it was time to move to a more clinically oriented cancer center.

While my husband understands the needs of my work and is totally supportive, he is a thoracic surgeon who was often on call and was for 20 years a department chair at M. D. Anderson; thus, he was not able to assume primary responsibility for the house or care of the children. Despite this, he did take his turn driving the kids to school when necessary and was more involved and available than most husbands of our generation. He was always helpful in a most positive manner. As his department grew and the kids were more independent, he did rearrange his schedule often to observe or participate in many events, especially during their high school years.

During the years of child-rearing responsibilities, I significantly decreased my travel and speaking engagements and did not pursue several leadership "promotion" possibilities. I admit that for approximately 10 years, I maintained steady forward momentum by keeping my grants, publishing papers, and graduating Ph.D. students but not taking serious risks in these areas. My challenges were in the areas of time and home management. Science advanced steadily but slowly in my lab, and probably not to the levels that would have been possible had I been childless. I now realize that I was distracted often by the daily needs of my family and struggled to compartmentalize home tasks at home and research tasks at the lab. Reading scientific papers at night and writing grants on the weekends had to be carefully planned and involved hiring a regular Saturday morning babysitter, enduring a lack of sleep, and/or skipping badly needed exercise. I did advance from associate professor to full professor and received an endowed Ashbel Smith Professorship during this time, so I was not considered to be slacking from the perspective of many. Now that our house is often empty, I am back in full gear: I'm receiving more local and international speaking invitations than I can possibly accept, serving on numerous study sections and many committees, and have received the first Francis King Black Memorial Professorship in Cancer Research. When I am in town, my daily life is spent in the office managing several major projects, which I supplement with Anusara yoga, pilates and aerobic exercise programs, attendance at concerts, and a variety of other social activities.

Now, Jack and I have had 30 wonderful years of marriage and raised two bright and beautiful daughters who are now young adults. I also must note that I am fortunate to have had several wonderful childcare helpers, including the same housekeeper, Maria Aviles Garcia, for all 22 years that we have lived in Houston; she and her family have become part of ours in many ways and hopefully will remain so. It has helped not only my husband and me but also my children to have an energetic adult who is available after school and whose sole purpose is to provide them with security and attention. According to my daughters, having another loving adult care for them after school has enriched their lives. Both my husband and I have been able to demonstrate to our daughters that with diligence and persistence, both men and women can succeed in their chosen careers *and* have a successful family life. In earlier years, usually when we arrived home, the children had been fed and homework was in the process of being done. In later years, we had dinner together if possible, as I tried to be home by 6 p.m. regularly. Rather than rushing home to cook dinner and get the children started on homework, we instead focused on relaxing with them and enjoying their company, helping with difficult homework problems or music practice, or attending one of their sports team activities.

In my life, I have consciously chosen to play three major roles. In the order of their development, they are: (1) professional cancer researcher, (2) wife, and (3) mother. My experience in all three of these roles has led me to two major conclusions. First, the early years must be managed optimally to achieve success in one's career. Then, if one chooses to, your life can be adjusted to accommodate marriage and a family. My belief is that the groundwork in the early years is *not* flexible, since periods of intense focus must be spent on obtaining the advanced degree, competing for early faculty positions and obtaining tenure. These tasks are immutable and consuming. The major selection for advancement in the academic field comes during this period. If you lose your focus and competitive position, it is extremely difficult, if not impossible, to catch up. Although I am certain that there are exceptions to this, I know of none. After the first grants and a tenured faculty position have been obtained, both men and women in research have a flexibility to accommodate family life and activities that those in many other professions would envy. Second, it is possible to have "everything" if that is what you want — but not all at once. In my view, it is hard for some young people today to delay gratification in some areas while they are establishing themselves in others. I believe that the only way to have both a family and a professional career is to acquire them sequentially, nurturing each in turn for a series of years before aiming for the next role.

My experience in mentoring also tells me that women, much more than men, strive to achieve the expectations of others. Women are not often aware of how to successfully balance their needs with the needs of the people who are attempting to influence them. Although statistics indicate that more women than men are graduating from college and then from medical and graduate schools, the higher ranks of academia remain filled primarily with men. Is this due to indecision or a lack of commitment on the part of women? Could it result from the diversion of women by family responsibilities? I do not know the answers to these questions, but I do advise women to stay true to themselves. I hope that by sharing my experiences and the way in which I have achieved my "everything," I will inspire the development of many more successful and happy women and men in science and medicine. Although I have had to overcome challenges, I am thankful for them, as they provided opportunities that made me a stronger person. With diligence, persistence, planning and confidence, you, too, can have your "everything." Best wishes to all of you!

Ellen R. Gritz, Ph.D.

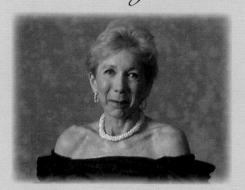

Professor and Chair of Behavioral Science
Olla S. Stribling Distinguished Chair
for Cancer Research

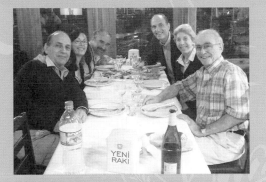

Ellen Gritz and husband Mickey Rosenau, at right, enjoy dinner with colleagues in Kusadasi, Turkey, in 2006 while Ellen was president of the Society for Research on Nicotine and Tobacco.

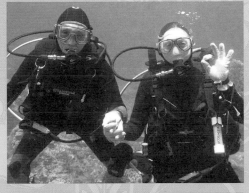

Mickey and Ellen had fun scuba diving off the coast of Sulanesi, Indonesia, in February 2005.

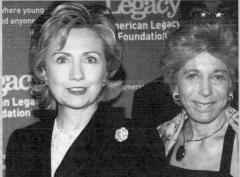

Ellen discussed health issues with Senator Hillary Rodham Clinton at an American Legacy Honors event in March 2006.

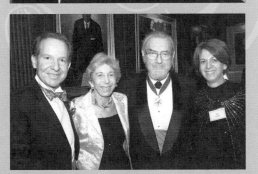

From left are Michael Fiore, M.D.; Ellen; former U.S. Surgeon General C. Everett Koop, M.D.; and Susan Curry, Ph.D., at Koop's 75th birthday gala in September 2006.

et's begin at the *end*, so to speak, which is *now*, with a really amazing event. I have just been elected to the Institute of Medicine, a branch of the National Academy of Sciences. Dr. John Mendelsohn, president of M. D. Anderson Cancer Center, has been the only IOM member at our institution; I have become the first woman faculty member to achieve this position. Did I *expect* this to happen? Not at all, which makes the honor and experience even more thrilling. Besides the personal feelings of accomplishment, what does this experience represent to me? As a psychologist trained in physiological, experimental and clinical psychology who has spent the majority of my career in comprehensive cancer centers, I am gratified by the acceptance of behavioral science as a mature career path and area of contribution to cancer research. Behavioral science is a *transdisciplinary* field — conducting research in cancer prevention and survivorship has led me into collaborations with colleagues in a variety of academic and medical disciplines, where all parties have been stimulated to learn much about each other's science. This integrative approach is the wave of the present *and* the future, and it is highly exciting to ride the crest.

I was raised in New York City, the grandchild of Eastern European immigrants fleeing the pogroms of the Czars and the child of parents who graduated from high school and then worked to support their elderly parents (in the case of my father) and male siblings who were attending college (in the case of my mother). I was the first in my immediate family to attend college. My younger brother was readily slated for medical school and is now a senior, community-based practicing radiologist. In my case, however, my parents envisioned me teaching elementary school. Nonetheless, my early ambition was to become a veterinarian, an interest that was probably stimulated by my love of animals, an affection with no known origin since our family apartment was too small for pets. While other girls read romance novels and Nancy Drew detective stories, I was studying cat and dog breeds and horse anatomy. I loved going to Madison Square Garden for the annual breed shows and equestrian competitions. The New York City school system had a special track for "gifted children," which advanced me rapidly. Thus, by high school I was two years younger than many of my classmates. I attended the Bronx High School of Science, where I further developed my love of biology and voluntarily headed the "animal squad," caring physically for the needs of a roomful of rats and mice, which I considered my pets. Sadly for me, many of them were used in scientific research and weren't around for very long.

By the time I got to Barnard College (women's college in the Columbia University system), my love of biology had led to a fascination with psychology and the brain. When I graduated in 1964 with a major in psychology, could

I have predicted my current career? Not at all — in fact, I had only the vaguest of career goals. I had always assumed that I would marry after college, stay home and raise children. However, nothing was further from the course that my life would actually take. In retrospect, attending a women's college provided well for my intellectual development and my initial flings at leadership (heading Barnard's upstate, rural camp site, among other extracurricular activities). However, even though Columbia College was directly across the street, at the time I would have preferred a coed school, since I enjoyed intellectual interaction with men. I certainly did encounter powerful women role models in the college leadership. In particular, President Millicent McIntosh stood out. She had earned a Ph.D. in English in 1926, raised five children, and served as Barnard's fourth president from 1947 to 1962. She inspired many undergraduates, including me, to set ambitious life goals.

When I graduated with honors from Barnard, I needed a break from intensive study, so I took a job at Bell Telephone Laboratories in Murray Hill, New Jersey. I had no help with finding this position. Rather, I found my job in *The New York Times* — literally. I spent an exhilarating two years at Bell Labs, a center of intellectual stimulation and pioneering research in communication. I learned computer programming in its most rudimentary forms (including machine language); made stereoscopic images for Dr. Bela Julesz, a famous scientist in the field of visual perception; and wrote a manual to teach FORTRAN, an early programming language. In addition to learning completely new fields in science, I started to mature emotionally, something that had been difficult to do living at home in Manhattan during my earlier schooling. I moved to New Jersey, was the first in my family to drive a car, had my own apartment, and joined the outing club, where I enjoyed white water canoeing, skiing, hiking and meeting like-minded souls.

At the end of two years at Bell Labs, my mentors there virtually propelled me to enroll in graduate school and suggested the brand new program at the University of California San Diego in La Jolla (UCSD). I received a full scholarship for the doctoral program and was in the first graduate class in psychology, where there were 12 professors and nine students. What an adventure — geographically, intellectually, emotionally and socially. The first six months that I lived in La Jolla, I floated along on a cloud, awed by the beauty of the Pacific Ocean, the tiny coastal towns, the opportunities to ski at Mammoth, hike in the Sierra Nevada, explore the desert, visit Mexico and swim daily in the ocean. Crowning the period was the incredible intellectual experience of having a very personalized graduate education led by a sterling group of professors, all of whom were also new to UCSD. I studied physiological psychology as a student of J. Anthony Deutsch, a brilliant scientist who guided me in work in the cholinergic mechanisms of rat and mouse memory. I wavered about applying to medical school and wondered whether my true calling was really medicine. I was able to participate in several classes at the new UCSD medical school, including gross anatomy and neurology, and also to study neuroscience at the Scripps Institute of Oceanography; this period was probably the foundation of my commitment to transdisciplinary education. In the end, I stuck with psychology and after receiving my doctoral degree, I was hired by my first true mentor, Murray Jarvik, M.D., Ph.D., a leader in research in memory and learning, especially in relation to psychoactive drugs.

Murray had the classical inquiring mind — he was inquisitive about everything, and in a most charming and endearing manner. When he hired me to run his new lab at the Veterans Administration Medical Center, West Los Angeles and UCLA, he was in the process of moving his research activities from the Albert Einstein College of Medicine in New York City. Thus, we started out fresh, researching memory and learning in drug-dependent humans, particularly those taking methadone, a synthetic opioid used to "maintain" opioid addicts, and naltrexone, an opioid receptor antagonist used to treat opioid and alcohol dependence. Frankly, I was happy to leave animal research and move on to human subjects, my ultimate interest. At the same time, Murray had a long fixation on cigarette smoking, which had originated when he observed chimpanzees appearing to smoke the cigarettes given them by their keepers at the Yerkes Primate Research Center. Murray was the first American scientist to establish that nicotine is the primary pharmacologic reinforcer in tobacco smoke. We and other gifted colleagues (Drs. Nina Schneider, Saul Shiffman and Jed Rose) spent several years examining the reinforcing properties of nicotine as well as studying drug withdrawal. Our laboratory was located in Brentwood, the psychiatric portion of the VA Hospital, where we had access to many patients with substance abuse diagnoses and chronic mental illness — and where almost all the patients smoked cigarettes.

In 1975, my life took another major turn (remember Yogi Berra's famous advice, "When you come to a fork in the road, take it.") I met my husband of now 32 years, Mickey Rosenau. I had always enjoyed outdoor activities, including swimming, hiking, tennis and scuba diving. Thus, I joined the Sierra Singles, a group dedicated to self-extinction. Soon afterwards, I went on a canoe trip on the Colorado River and met Mickey, whom I would marry six months to the day later. Needless to say, we hit it off instantly, he proposed that very same day, and we were married in the presence of aging relatives and numerous friends on a beautiful lawn in Pacific Palisades, California, overlooking the Pacific Ocean. Mickey had been married previously and had a daughter 11 years younger than me. The next year she graduated from college and married, and we became grandparents in the course of good time (I call it "skip generation" grand-parenting). We did not have children of our own, which permitted us a great deal of freedom in career development, travel, and the evolution of our own mature interests in culture, the arts and global conservation.

After Mickey and I married, we each took a big step in developing our respective careers. Mickey, who has a background in engineering physics, had worked for sophisticated technology companies, first in a scientific and then in a managerial capacity. He wanted to set up his own business as a management consultant and leave the corporate world. My having a full-time academic position allowed him to do that, from a start-up status, quite successfully. Following that year, I, too, decided to fulfill my career ambitions in clinical psychology. I cut back on my research position to take the necessary classes in the graduate clinical psychology program at the University of Southern California, achieving licensure in 1979. At that point, I faced a decision about whether to leave research and seek a full-time clinical position or whether to combine the two. The lure of research remained too strong, so I established a part-time private practice for the next several years to satisfy my desire to be a psychotherapist. My primary appointment was still at the VA, where I was now chief of the Human Behavioral Pharmacology and Psychosocial Research Laboratory, and I had recently been promoted to associate professor at UCLA in the Research Series.

A major career opportunity arose in 1979, when I was invited to write the behavioral section of the first Report of the Surgeon General on Women and Smoking. That landmark 1980 report signaled the beginning of a 21-year association with the National Office on Smoking and Health and editorship on 10 Surgeon General's reports, with several remarkable colleagues who remain good friends to this day (Dr. David Burns, Don Shopland and John Pinney). That experience led me to many national leadership opportunities in tobacco research and tobacco control at the National Institutes of Health and other organizations.

Also about that time, I began to realize that I wanted a closer affiliation at UCLA, particularly with the UCLA Jonsson Comprehensive Cancer Center (JCCC). Dr. Joseph Cullen, a psychologist who became a major figure in cancer control later at the National Cancer Institute (NCI), recruited me in 1981 to be the director of the Macomber-Murphy Cancer Prevention Program at the JCCC. Joe was another significant mentor who realized the critical role of tobacco in cancer prevention. My interest in women and smoking would gradually expand to other special populations, including medical patients and cancer patients in particular. Joe died suddenly and tragically of a brain tumor a number of years later, but he still looms large in the history of cancer control. I was honored to be the first recipient of the

Joseph W. Cullen Memorial Lectureship Award from the American Society of Preventive Oncology (ASPO) in 1992.

Another life-changing event was my husband's diagnosis with testicular cancer in 1981. This was long before Lance Armstrong made that disease a household name but, fortunately, quite soon after Dr. Larry Einhorn developed the famous "Einhorn regimen" of cisplatin, bleomycin, and vinblastine, which raised the cure rate from about 10 percent to over 90 percent. My husband's illness and curative treatment course (surgery plus chemotherapy) lasted less than six months but was to change the entire course of my professional life as well as strengthen our marriage significantly through trial by fire. I became much more interested in the psychosocial aspects of cancer treatment and survivorship and found a focus for applying my clinical psychology training and licensure to research and patient care. Indeed, several years later, I was awarded a grant from the American Cancer Society, California Division, to study the long-term effects of testicular cancer on individuals and couples, and, from this grant, a series of landmark papers were published. My husband and I vowed to live by the principle of *carpe diem*, and we have made quality of life and balance in our professional and personal relationships a hallmark of our lives together, one that has been ever more nourishing and replenishing.

I became a full-time faculty member at UCLA in 1984, bringing my career at the VA to an end. Over the next two years, I had two more outstanding mentors, Helene Brown and Dr. Lester Breslow. They served as the joint directors of the Division of Cancer Control at the JCCC between the time when Joe Cullen departed for the NCI in 1984 and the point when I became director in 1986. Lester, a giant in the field of cancer prevention and public health, taught me the value of having respect for all colleagues, particularly junior colleagues. He advocated hiring people smarter than oneself and letting them shine. That principle reflects well upon a leader. I still try to follow his advice. Helene Brown served as a role model of generosity and human relationships. She was an "oncopolitician," as she termed it. Helene had been a national leader in the American Cancer Society and was well versed in the role of the voluntary health organizations in cancer prevention and control, serving on many advisory committees at the NCI and other organizations. She outshone anyone I had known in the ability to care about every person in our organization and to show that generosity through frequent contact, personal communication and the expression of thanks for accomplishments. These critical qualities of leadership — recognizing the value of your faculty and staff and expressing your praise and appreciation — have served me well throughout my career.

As I became more active in cancer control and tobacco research, I developed a collegial base of behavioral scientists who were now also leaders in similar types of research activities across the nation. Through this network of friends and colleagues, I came to understand that my academic career, in terms of rank and compensation, was significantly behind that of my peers. I can only say now that I was naive and idealistic in not pressing for advancement and higher pay earlier. What held me back was my modesty and belief that since my husband had a flourishing business, we were not in critical need of more income. Is this a typical woman's belief? It may have been then, but certainly it is not now — I hope! Seeking rewards more commensurate with my career stage, I applied for positions and received a very good offer from another university. However, I chose to remain at UCLA. I was promoted to full professor and received a change in university faculty series and a significant increase in salary. The new academic appointment was in Head and Neck Surgery, headed by Dr. Paul Ward, where I became a professor in residence. Dr. Ward, a visionary leader and teacher of surgeons, believed that behavioral science significantly enhanced the existing programs in basic science and clinical medicine in his department. This appointment was another transdisciplinary experience in my career, one that I dearly loved. It included clinical psychotherapy practice with cancer patients as well as the research I had been conducting with colleagues in surgery and maxillofacial prosthodontics. Our smoking cessation study in this cancer patient population was another landmark in the literature.

My final career relocation came in 1993, when M. D. Anderson Cancer Center recruited me to found the first academic department of behavioral science in any comprehensive cancer center in the nation, a status it retains to this day. I can honestly say that I was bowled over by M. D. Anderson — its vision and mission, size, structure, patient population, clinical and research opportunities, and outstanding faculty. I was simultaneously looking at several other positions, but M. D. Anderson won, hands down. My husband had the flexibility to move his management consulting firm at will, so relocation was not a significant barrier for him. We were unusual in that respect: moving spouses, particularly male spouses, is often a deal breaker for senior women faculty. We sold our house in Los Angeles and moved to Houston over the Memorial Day weekend in 1993, accompanied by our aging cat, Sasha. We lived in an apartment while we built a contemporary home, another dream we fulfilled. Outside, a large garden and my 100-plus orchids in their greenhouse connect us to nature daily. Along the years, after Sasha passed away, we adopted Tenzing PurrBall and Lady Godiva, two adorable and eccentric kitties.

I have spent the past 14 years at M. D. Anderson building and developing my own research program as well as the Department of Behavioral Science. Beginning with one faculty position (mine), the department has grown to 24 faculty (in tenure and non-tenure series) and a total workforce of more than

100. My own research in smoking prevention and cessation has continued, most recently adding a new population of interest: persons living with HIV/ AIDS. This group has more than doubled the smoking prevalence of the general public (50 percent versus 21 percent) and can derive important and potentially life-saving benefits from stopping smoking. Other research programs that I have developed since coming to M. D. Anderson include skin cancer prevention through sun protection interventions among healthy pre-school children and in families of melanoma survivors; psychosocial aspects of genetic testing and counseling for hereditary non-polyposis colon cancer; and a prospective study of neurocognitive function in testicular cancer patients treated with high-dose chemotherapy. This last study was the first grant awarded by the Lance Armstrong Foundation, and thus it has had special meaning for me.

Even more meaningful than the maturation and expansion of my own career and research accomplishments have been the satisfaction and pride gained from the successful development of my department. Being a department chair at this dynamic institution is challenging, demanding and gratifying. Mentoring postdoctoral students, young faculty and new faculty as they come to our cancer center is an ongoing and consequential role. Putting behavioral science on the academic map of a cancer center requires demonstrating the value of our work and its transdisciplinary connections to the basic and clinical sciences and to other fields in the population sciences. Our scientific accomplishments involve changing behavior: reducing risk factors in healthy community-dwelling persons, designing strategies for those at elevated risk for cancer as well as those with cancer, and improving quality of life of patients and survivors. Disseminating effective interventions and reaching underserved populations is a high-priority aspect of behavioral science research.

Another intensely rewarding leadership activity at M. D. Anderson is the Faculty Health Committee. In 2001, two colleagues (Drs. Georgia Thomas, chief of Employee Health, and Walter Baile, section chief of Psychiatry at that time) and I conceptualized a faculty health program that would focus on prevention of burnout and distress, promoting work-life balance and introducing a range of wellness activities into faculty programming. We undertook this initiative with the full support of Dr. Mendelsohn and the other M. D. Anderson senior leadership following the tragic suicide of a physician colleague. Over the past seven years, along with a strong committee and institutional resources, we have built a multidimensional and vibrant program, which now has a full-time director in a faculty position in my department. The program includes: a completely confidential and free psychotherapy resource outside M. D. Anderson that is available to faculty and immediate family for assessment, brief intervention and referral;

numerous lectures and seminars on topics related to stress, burnout and wellness; a range of experiential programs on topics such as meditation, mental fitness and work-life balance; and education for faculty leaders on how to recognize and deal with distressed or potentially impaired faculty. A strong aspect of the program involves its sponsorship of periodic artistic performances. These have included an annual piano concert and lecture delivered by a well-known musician/psychiatrist and focused on the life of a great composer who had a significant mental or physical illness; a concert of opera arias and duets exemplifying illness and death, performed by Houston Grand Opera studio artists and narrated by accomplished interpreters of the history of opera and operatic music; jazz performances; and upcoming dance recitals. Not only has leading this program been a tremendous pleasure for me personally, but also I feel I have made an important contribution to my colleagues and to the institution in this role.

I have received a variety of meaningful honors and awards in the course of my career. Serving as both the president of the American Society of Preventive Oncology, from 1993 to 1995, and the president of my professional organization, the Society for Research in Nicotine and Tobacco, from 2006 to 2007, had provided incredibly important and enjoyable experiences, allowing me to exert some personal degree of leadership in my discipline. At M. D. Anderson, I have received the James W. Elkins Faculty Achievement Award in Cancer Prevention, the Business and Professional Women's Award of Texas, and three endowed positions: the Annie Laurie Howard Research Professorship, the Frank T. McGraw Memorial Chair in the Study of Cancer, and most recently (2005) the Olla S. Stribling Distinguished Chair for Cancer Research. Finally, election to the Institute of Medicine in October 2007 has been immensely gratifying.

Throughout my career, achieving a balance between work and personal life has been a high priority, strongly reinforced by my husband's experience with cancer 27 years ago. Together we have explored the natural world, traveling widely, hiking three times in the Himalayas (in Nepal, Bhutan and Sikkim), and scuba diving across the Asia-Pacific (in the Maldives, Philippines, Malaysia, Solomon Islands and many times in Indonesia, our favorite destination). We are active in Houston's cultural and artistic offerings. I am a devoted opera aficionado and sit on the Board of Trustees of the Houston Grand Opera. We attend and support ballet, modern dance, chamber music, the Museum of Fine Arts and the Houston Zoo. Personally, I swim 1.5 miles daily, which keeps both my mind and body in shape. While my dad passed away from prostate cancer in 1991, my mother is in excellent health and celebrated her 100th birthday in 2008. I hope that I can follow in her footsteps!

Kelly K. Hunt, M.D.

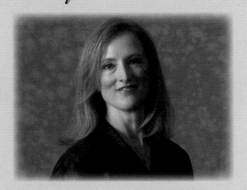

Professor of Surgical Oncology

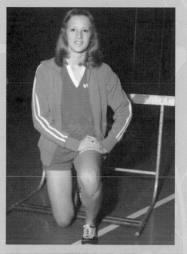

Kelly was getting ready for competition as a member of her high school track team in 1980.

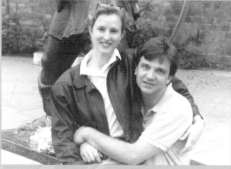

Kelly and husband Steve Swisher, M.D., enjoyed outings while taking their surgical training in Nottingham, England, in 1991.

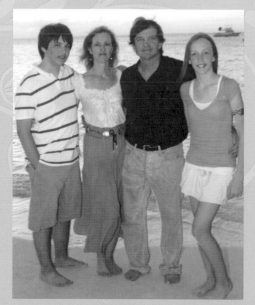

Son Chris and daughter Shannon pose with their parents Kelly and Steve during a family vacation in 2007 to the Turks and Caicos Islands.

In my current role as a professor of surgery and chief of the Surgical Breast Service at M. D. Anderson Cancer Center, I have the privilege of caring for patients who not only are dealing with the physical effects of receiving several types of treatment simultaneously but also are struggling with the emotional trauma of having a life-threatening illness. Working with patients and families who confront such heavy issues of life and death on a daily basis helps keep my own life and career in perspective. Just when I start to feel sorry for myself because of the demands of my career, I witness a young man with bone cancer who has a prosthetic limb and who is having difficulty walking from the parking lot to the clinic for his appointment. Such things, viewed nearly every day, serve as a wake-up call that helps keep me focused on what is important.

Working in a comprehensive cancer center allows me to pursue both clinical and translational research programs while also maintaining a busy surgical practice. I spend about 50 percent of my time taking care of patients with breast cancer and other soft tissue malignant tumors; the rest of my time is divided between clinical and translational research, teaching and administration. Dividing my time this way works well to keep me engaged because, just when things start to get tough in the clinic, some exciting new piece of data emerges in the laboratory. Similarly, when things become frustrating in the lab, I can turn my focus to clinical care and try to affect a patient's life through surgical and medical interventions. Thus, the blend of clinical and research duties provides an ideal work mix, allowing me to remain energized and focused on the task at hand, namely, fighting cancer.

Entering the medical profession was hardly a sudden decision for me; in fact, I can remember telling people that I was going to be a doctor ever since I was in the first grade. Of course, back then I had no idea of what was involved in terms of the years required for education and training or of the sacrifices that I would have to make in my personal life. I was born in a very small town in Montana and am the middle child, with two older brothers and a younger sister. We were very close in age but had very different interests and talents. We moved every few years due to my father's employment in the retail business. I was always up for the adventure of a new town and a new school, but it was very tough on my mother, who had to move our entire household so many times, often on very short notice. My parents were always extremely supportive of my goals and never told me that I should or should not pursue a particular career. Our family life was very traditional. My mother was a homemaker who did all of the cooking and cleaning and even made all of our clothes. My father was in the retail business and worked such long hours that we usually only saw him on Sundays. I knew that both of my parents worked extremely hard, but I really only saw my mother in action. She gave my sister and me typical chores for young girls, such as cleaning up after dinner and doing the laundry. Meanwhile, my brothers were expected to take out the trash and occasionally help with the yard work. I wasn't really upset about the differences in the workload, but I do remember thinking that the boys should be able to clean and cook just as well as I could. And I thought that I should be able to drive the tractor and mow the lawn as well as they could. Why were there gender-specific tasks anyway? Nevertheless, both my mother and father set good examples for my siblings and me. For this reason, I always felt that "if you worked hard, you could succeed and achieve your goals." I believe that this mindset prepared me for a challenging career in surgery and academic medicine, but I would later encounter many people who carried the old gender-specific stereotypes beyond the home and into education and even into the profession of medicine.

From an early age, I enjoyed school work and had an inquisitive nature. When I was 4 years old, I watched my brothers leave for school in the morning and begged my mother to let me go with them. I wasn't satisfied to stay at home and play; I wanted to go out and explore. I enjoyed science and math in school but did not have any role models to show me how I might apply these studies to a career. My high school required all female students to take home economics. I already knew how to cook and sew, but I did not see how these things were going to prepare me for a career. I continued to think about becoming a physician but saw very few examples of women in medicine, so I was uncertain of how to proceed if I planned to have a career and a family.

After graduating from high school in Memphis, Tennessee, I chose to stay there for college as well. This was mostly for family reasons, but I think I was also a bit weary from the frequent moves during my childhood. As a freshman in college, I did not declare a major, but I did follow a premed curriculum. I finally decided to pursue a major in physical chemistry with a minor in mathematics. It was in the chemistry department that I first encountered professors who were less than enthusiastic about having a female student in their classes. I worked very hard and excelled in all of my classes and laboratories. Despite the fact that I had an A+ average in advanced physical chemistry, one of my professors was very cold to me and refused to acknowledge me in class. These were small classes, so the lack of interaction was quite obvious. One day, I mustered all my courage and went to his office to ask for help with a problem set that he had assigned. He was so rude to me that I finally asked him why he treated me so dismissively. He said that he didn't understand why I wanted to pursue these studies and that he did not feel it was a suitable career for women. I broke down and cried as I realized that the ability to succeed might depend on factors that were out of my control. It did not seem fair that even with a lot of hard work and determination, the fact that I was a woman might affect my chances to succeed. The experience with my chemistry professor helped me understand that not everyone would be supportive of my goals and that it was up to me to seek out supportive mentors. Fortunately, another professor offered me a research elective in his laboratory, where I worked on geometric isomerism. This experience sparked my interest in a research career. The freedom to question, to create, and even to fail was exciting and fueled my desire to become a research investigator.

Although I probably would have been very happy pursuing a career in chemistry and basic research, I still had an interest in medicine and patient care. I had always enjoyed working with people, and the challenge of getting into medical school and becoming a physician intrigued me. I applied to medical schools with a backup plan to pursue a master's degree in chemistry if I did not get in. When I interviewed at different medical schools, I was asked many questions about how I would manage a career *and* a family. Did I plan to have children? Since my father was not a doctor, did I really know what I was getting into? I interviewed at a number of schools around the country but found that the University of Tennessee in Memphis had all of the elements I was searching for: a broad variety of clinical experiences and a large medical center with the opportunity for involvement in patient care activities very early in the curriculum. Once I was accepted into medical school, I found that the curriculum was indeed demanding. The sheer volume of knowledge we were expected to assimilate was daunting, but I was determined to make it and was not going to fail. I loved gross anatomy and was very meticulous with my dissections. One of the instructors suggested that I might pursue a surgical specialty, but I had no idea what that meant or what it would entail. At that time, only a few women were on the medical school faculty, and *none* specialized in surgery.

As a third-year student, I rotated through the general surgery service and noted that there were only a few female residents and that they did not seem very happy. Furthermore, none of these women were married or had children. I was very motivated to have a successful career, but I also wanted to have a family. I remember thinking that if I was going to become a surgeon, I would probably never have children. When I spoke to my advisor about pursuing surgery as a specialty, he told me that I would need to take an elective with one of the senior surgical faculty and impress him with my knowledge and skills so that I could get a strong letter of recommendation for my residency applications. I liked the fast pace of the surgical service and did not mind the long hours. I was, however, unprepared for the reaction of some of the attending surgeons whenever I discussed my plans to pursue a surgical career. One of the attending transplant surgeons told me to bail out and look for something that would give me more "personal time." Since

I was a good student and very hard working, I did not understand why the faculty were not more encouraging. As the time neared for me to apply for residency training, I remained unsure of a specialty and wondered whether I should consider medicine or pediatrics. Toward the end of my surgical elective, however, as I was making rounds with one of the senior surgeons, he said something that finally gave me the encouragement I needed. While removing the dressing from the incision in one of his post-op patients, he commented to the patient that he had always thought there were two places that women did not belong: the golf course and the operating room. He then paused and added, "I think I might have been wrong, at least about the second one." Although he was not talking *to* me, I decided that he was talking *about* me, and that was all the encouragement that I needed to forge ahead.

While most of the medical students in my class planned to remain in the southeast for their residency training, I sent applications to general surgery programs all over the country. When I visited programs on the west coast and the east coast, I was encouraged to find a few more women who were upper-level residents, and some of them even seemed to be enjoying themselves. I was particularly interested in the "seven-year" programs that allowed for two years of dedicated research time in the third and fourth postgraduate years. I was matched with the University of California-Los Angeles, where I was one of eight first-year residents (six men and two women). That first year was especially challenging since most of the surgical services required residents to take calls in the hospital every other night or to take calls from home every night. Many times I wondered if I could physically do the work and still have time to read about surgical diseases. Fortunately, the other residents in the program were extremely supportive and, overall, we had a great time despite being chronically sleep deprived. The program had recently changed from a pyramidal system in which many good residents were eliminated each year to one in which a spot was guaranteed to eight categorical residents. Nevertheless, we were still haunted by stories about residents being fired because they were a few minutes late for rounds or because they didn't have a patient's lab results memorized whenever an attending physician called (any time of the day or night). Regardless of how hard we worked, we didn't receive much positive feedback, so we joked that "if the attending physicians weren't yelling at you, you were probably doing a good job." Darwin would have been proud of our surgical training system.

It was during my research years that I met and married my husband Steve. We were actually in the same intern class but had very few interactions during our clinical rotations in the first two years of our training. He tells me that he thought I was very intense and intimidating. During our research time, we were in neighboring laboratories and would see each other at weekly lab meetings and research conferences. I guess I seemed more relaxed to him in the research setting because he would often drop by to talk and discuss research. Even though we worked long hours in the laboratory, it seemed very easy because we were free of any clinical responsibilities. This allowed us to pursue our research interests and still have time to do things outside the hospital. We found that we shared many interests in common and decided to get married at the end of our research years before we went back to our clinical rotations.

Once we resumed our clinical rotations, things became quite challenging. We were always on different services and rarely had any time off together, but we tried to support each other as much as possible. When we were senior residents, we decided it was time to start a family. Although many people thought we were crazy, we were excited about having children but really couldn't determine an ideal time to get started. We met with our department chair to discuss the possibility, and he was completely at a loss about how to advise us. Hospital policy addressed neither the issue of maternity leave for surgical residents nor the very specific requirements as to how much time residents could be out during their chief year and still qualify to take their boards. By this time I was already well into my pregnancy, and my department chair said he would treat me as if I had a broken arm or some other physical impairment that would require me to be out for a period of time. To add insult to injury, the other female resident in the same year of the program was pregnant at the same time. I think we actually planned it this way because we figured that there was no way they would fire both of us. She and I were able to cross-cover for each other on our clinical services, which allowed us to each take about six weeks off to be at home with our newborns. Seeing two pregnant chief residents obviously had a big impact on the medical students interviewing for the UCLA residency program that year because six of the eight first-year residents who matched with the program that following year were women. Not all the faculty was supportive. One faculty member actually told me that he thought we needed to put birth control pills in the water! Having a newborn baby while also trying to meet the demands of being a surgical chief resident was an immense challenge. I felt like I was always in the wrong place at the wrong time and often doubted whether I was a good mother *or* a good chief resident. Fortunately, Steve was very supportive, and we were also able to find a nanny to help watch our son, Christopher, during the day. Even though Steve always assured me that I was doing a great job as both a mom and a surgeon, I still felt unsure about this.

After finishing our surgical residencies at UCLA, Steve decided that he wanted to pursue a career in thoracic surgical oncology, which required his becoming a cardiothoracic surgery resident at M. D. Anderson Cancer Center. This was not optimal for me because I had been offered a surgical oncology faculty position at UCLA, but M. D. Anderson did not want to offer me a faculty position unless I completed a surgical oncology fellowship at M. D. Anderson. Since Steve was so committed to becoming a thoracic surgical oncologist, I decided to accept the M. D. Anderson surgical oncology fellowship. In the long run, things ultimately worked out, but I was somewhat upset about having to become a fellow again even though I already had a surgical oncology faculty position at UCLA. To make things more challenging, we were expecting our second child, Shannon, at the end of June, just before I had to start my fellowship in Houston. Fortunately, we convinced the obstetrician to induce labor a few weeks early and, after I had delivered a healthy baby girl, we moved our family to Houston.

Even though we had already successfully raised our son Chris during my chief resident year at UCLA, the challenges of having two children, living in a new city and trying to complete two fellowships often was difficult. As fellows, we did not have much control over our time, and we also had many financial burdens. Because we were planning for academic careers, we were both pursuing research projects, which made it difficult to spend an adequate amount of time with our children. Luckily, my mother lived nearby, and we also had a very supportive nanny who spent many hours helping us raise our small children. I am not really certain how our marriage survived this very busy and complicated time in our lives, but I like to think it is because neither Steve nor I expected the other to do anything that we would not do ourselves, either at home or at work. Whoever was at home with the kids would cook, clean, do the laundry and try to fill in for the missing parent. As a result, our children were happy and healthy, and we were both able to fulfill our clinical responsibilities, present our research at national meetings, and publish papers.

Following completion of our surgical residencies, our next hurdle was to find faculty positions that would allow both of us to pursue our clinical interests and develop our research programs. We each knew what we wanted to do; the questions were whether we would both have the opportunity to pursue our goals and how we would decide who would give up what in order to keep our family together. We were each invited for interviews at several institutions across the country and anticipated that we would ultimately return to California, where we had great mentors and a network of family and friends. However, we were incredibly fortunate to be offered faculty positions at M. D. Anderson, which allowed us to remain in Houston and each pursue tenure track positions as clinician investigators. Now my biggest problem was trying to manage my time between clinical practice, research and family life. I felt like a kid in a candy store with so many great opportunities — and I wanted them all! My training in surgical oncology was broad, and I wanted to keep my clinical skills sharp in different areas to keep all my options open. This meant that I had clinics in multiple centers and was always running from one place to another. My department chair once commented that I seemed to flourish in a state of dynamic tension. I didn't really like being so harried and hurried, but I was excited about the progress of my research, and my clinical practice was challenging and stimulating. Though one of the female faculty was openly disapproving of my efforts and commented that she thought I should be more focused, my department chair, in contrast, was very supportive of my clinical and research endeavors and put me up for early promotion. In fact, he asked me what I wanted to do and how he could help me achieve my goals. This made me think back to the earlier years of my training, when I had experienced some prejudice from male professors. Things had definitely changed!

I am frequently asked by female residents and students how best to balance career and family. Communication has been the key in my family. My husband and I are constantly calling and e-mailing each other to be certain we are on the same page with what is happening at home and at work. We both travel a lot, and we often take one or both of our children with us even if they have to miss a few days of school. Recently, my daughter and I were out walking our two dogs when she commented how much she loves her life. She even said that I was a "cool mom." That was really a defining moment for me because I have often felt guilty about not being the homemaker that my mother was, and I often worry that my busy career might somehow be a disadvantage to my children.

Finally, I believe that there is nothing wrong with wanting it all, but in successfully pursuing that path, we need to be happy with the choices we make and not worry about what others think. With dedication, focus and hard work, it is possible to successfully balance family priorities with those of a career in academic medicine. We all have different talents, and if we share them, we can definitely make this world a better place.

Eugenie S. Kleinerman, M.D.

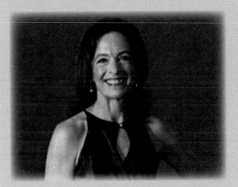

Professor and Head of Division of Pediatrics
Mosbacher Pediatrics Chair

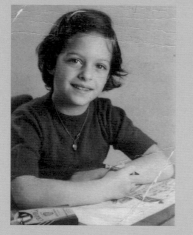

Genie, age 5, liked kindergarten at Moreland Elementary School in Shaker Heights, Ohio.

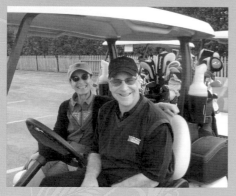

Genie joined husband Leonard Zwelling, M.D., for the Department of Chaplaincy and Pastoral Education's annual golf tournament in 2006.

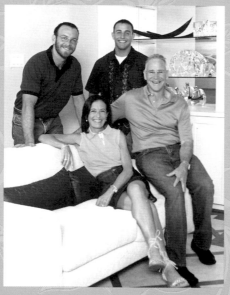

Sons Richard, standing at left, and Andrew posed at home with Genie and Leonard, in 2006.

(Photo courtesy of Britt Redding Associates)

was always the smallest or next to the smallest in my class. Growing up in the '50s with my petite form, wavy brown hair and name "Genie Sue," no one took me seriously when I declared that I wanted to be a physician. "No honey," they would say as they patted me on the head, "you mean you want to be a nurse. You're too cute to be a doctor." This made me boil inside.

I was inspired by my father, who was an academic physician, and by my pediatrician, whom I regarded as the most caring, funny and dedicated human being on earth. Those were the days of house calls, and as a close friend of my father's (they practiced in the same hospital), Dr. Mortimor frequented our home for both business and social reasons. Measles, chicken pox, rubella, strep throat, fevers — he was there with a joke, a funny voice, a calm soothing hand and reassuring words for my mother. I was devastated when the University of New Mexico recruited him away to be their chief of pediatrics. How could anyone be as good as he?

My dad, of course, thought that medicine was "the only occupation" and was proud, thrilled and supportive of my plan to be a physician. My mother, a woman who preached equal opportunity for women before it was in vogue, was even more encouraging. "You need to have goals of your own, an identity of your own, achievements of your own," she would tell my two sisters and me. She had left graduate school to marry my father and on some level clearly regretted not completing her master's degree. In high school, I excelled in biology and won a "Future Scientist of America" contest. Surely now, I thought, people would see that I was serious.

I arrived at Washington University in 1967 and promptly made an appointment with the pre-med advisor, Dean W., who was, to my delight, a woman. Strangely, she did not pay much attention during the appointment, and I could tell that she, like many others, did not take me seriously. During my undergraduate years, she made it clear that she thought medicine was not in my future. I was a sorority girl, a cheerleader, participated in Greek sing and campus musicals, and was a finalist for homecoming queen in my junior year. How could I expect people to believe that I had the required dedication and stamina for a medical career? I remember boiling inside yet again and thinking, "But my male pre-med classmates are in fraternities, play sports, and get drunk and high every weekend. Does that bring *their* dedication into question?"

So, on my own I filled out my applications, took the MCATs, scheduled medical school interviews, and did not request a letter of recommendation from Dean W. Fortunately, since my father was an academic physician, he could help and advise me — that is, when I would listen. You cannot imagine my excitement when I was accepted to Duke Medical School, my dream school. In August 1971, I boarded an airplane with my microscope in hand and flew down to the wilds of Durham, North Carolina, scared but excited and elated.

The campus was every bit as beautiful as I remembered it from when I had visited in eighth grade. My fellow students were friendly and supportive. The small class size (115 with 15 women) allowed us to get to know each other rather quickly. The schedule was grueling, as the Duke curriculum crammed all the basic science courses into year one. Year two was spent doing the required clinical rotations. This allowed Duke medical students to either do research or take advanced graduate courses in year three. This option would prove to be of enormous benefit to me by providing outstanding research training that shaped my career. During that first year, we went to class from 8 a.m. to 5 p.m. Monday through Friday and from 8 a.m. until noon on Saturday. Sunday was spent in the library. Anatomy was particularly challenging as the vocabulary was all new and I felt like I was looking up every other word in my medical dictionary. Nevertheless, it was exciting, challenging and also fun. During that first month, I met with my medical school advisor, Dr. R., a pediatric oncologist to whom I was assigned since I wanted to be a pediatrician. As I made my way through the hospital to his office, I was excited, thinking "Certainly this time I'll have access to a mentor."

That turned out be to wishful thinking! Dr. R. was cold and tight-lipped and asked me no questions. I finally broke the silence and inquired whether I had done something to offend him. "No," he responded. "I just don't think women belong in medicine." I couldn't believe my ears. How could this same thing be happening to me again? I shyly asked why he thought women didn't belong in medicine. He responded, "because they get married or pregnant and drop out of residency programs, putting hardships on the remaining residents." He then proceeded to relate two more anecdotes. Just this year, one of the pediatric residents had gotten pregnant, developed complications, had to go on bed rest and had left the program. As a result, the hospital was short-staffed and the remaining residents were stressed. A few years earlier, one of the female residents had transferred to another program because she had gotten married and her husband was doing a residency elsewhere. I don't know how I got the nerve, but I then asked Dr. R., "Have you ever had male residents who left the program?" "Yes," he said. When I asked what their reasons for leaving were, he replied, "Well, one had a nervous breakdown, and the other was dismissed because he was incompetent."

I sat in disbelief, thinking to myself, "Well, I guess (in his view) being incompetent or having a nervous breakdown is preferable to leaving due to pregnancy complications or marriage." That was the end of my appointment, and I never saw Dr. R. again during my four years at Duke.

My 14 female classmates were all amazing individuals. We all recognized the burden on our shoulders. We were being watched. We would be tested. Were we really serious and could we stand up to the grueling schedule and tough "on-your-feet grilling" that goes on during clinical rotations? We had heard that the chief of surgery would never take a woman into his residency program. The Obstetrics-Gynecology program had taken only one or two. In retrospect, it was a fascinating time and exciting to be a part of the change that was taking place. Fittingly, the chief of surgery finally did take a woman into his residency program, and that woman was from my class.

Year two proved to have its own challenges. The call schedule for internal medicine was five nights a week. Unfortunately, there were no on-call rooms for women, which necessitated my leaving the hospital to go home to sleep when I could. Unlike the male medical students on service with me, quick naps in the on-call room were not an option. One late night as I was finishing up with my charts, I looked around to find the ward empty. There were no interns or residents, and the other student with me on the rotation (a male) was not there. "Oh well," I thought, "finish up and go get a few hours of sleep at home." As I was exiting the hospital, I walked by the cafeteria, and there, sitting around the table were the two interns, the junior and senior residents, the other medical student, and the chief resident, having midnight coffee rounds. I found out the next day from the other student that this informal gathering was by invitation only. So, I had not forgotten or failed to listen. I was simply not included! But by this time, I had stopped boiling inside when these things happened. Instead, I just shook my head and shrugged it off.

Lest you think that I had only negative experiences at Duke Medical School, let me quickly shift the focus to the attending physician. Dr. Ralph Snyderman was a young faculty member recruited from the National Institutes of Health who was doing research in rheumatology and inflammation. It was fortunate for me that he was the attending during my internal medicine rotation. An animated, enthusiastic teacher, he convinced me to come to his lab to do immunology research in my third year. Next to marrying my husband (whom I met during the first month of year one in medical school and married at the end of year one), this was the best decision I have ever made. It changed my life, started me on a new path, and shaped my thinking as an investigator. Dr. Snyderman taught me to design experiments, to interpret data and to write. I learned how to put together an abstract, a 10-minute platform talk and a scientific manuscript. Many Saturdays were spent writing and rewriting our manuscripts, and to this day I still borrow some of the verbiage we used back then. He was my first mentor, and I owe much of my inspiration and success to him. Under his direction, my research career was born. During that year in his laboratory, I presented at the National Federation Meeting, was interviewed on a local

TV show, "At Home With Peggy Mann," published three papers, and won a national competition. At my medical school graduation, I received the Sandoz Award for Meritorious Original Student Research. This was an amazing moment for me.

I did my pediatric residency at the Children's Hospital National Medical Center in Washington, D.C., since my husband had been accepted as a clinical associate in the Medicine Branch at the National Cancer Institute (NCI). I had ruled out the Johns Hopkins residency program for me, as it was in Baltimore and had an every-other-night call schedule. I didn't think my marriage would survive the schedule and the commute. During those three years of intense clinical exposure, however, I decided that I missed the research, so I applied for and was accepted as a clinical associate in the Metabolism Branch of the NCI, a position that included one clinical and two research years. At the end of my second year, our first son, Richard, was born, and it was then that the reality of being a working mother, with its guilt and torn commitment, hit me. When Richard was a year old, I transitioned to a faculty position at the Frederick Cancer Research facility, 30 miles north of our home in Potomac, Maryland. My husband continued his position at the NCI in Bethesda. My commute was against traffic, but the hour-long drive each way added to the challenges of being a working mother. Carpooling for nursery school was impossible, as was the option to pop out for an hour or so to see the Halloween pageant or get to a teacher conference or school program. But I had an excellent nanny and never worried about Richard's safety or whether he was being cared for. My greatest fear was that he wouldn't know that I was his mother!

In Frederick, Maryland, I had the great fortune of meeting my second mentor, Dr. Josh Fidler, who shaped and influenced my most productive years as a scientist. Even more significant, he let me know that family was the most important priority. He pointed out that while balancing work and motherhood was difficult, I would be shortchanging myself if I didn't do both. Richard was 4 when we followed Dr. Fidler to M. D. Anderson Cancer Center. This was the third best decision of my life.

Houston and M. D. Anderson proved to be the right places at the right time in my life, for professional and personal reasons. Two years after we arrived, my second son, Andrew, was born, adding additional challenges and guilt but enormous joy. One never escapes the "guilty mother" syndrome of trying to be all things to all people, both at work and at home. In managing this situation, there is no substitute for a supportive spouse, an encouraging mentor who advocates for you, a wonderful community with resources and friends who will pitch in and help, and strong support staff at work. An efficient administrative assistant, nurse, or laboratory technician can make all the difference. Look for and recruit such individuals, and be good to them. They can lessen the wrinkles in your hectic days. I have tried to pass on these lessons to women medical students, graduate students and junior faculty. I let them know that they are not alone in their struggle with guilt as working mothers; that a persona combining determination, focus and poise scores more points with our male colleagues; and, most important, that family relationships are key. Turning down an international speaking invitation, a seminar, or a committee appointment or publishing one less paper will not torpedo your career. My favorite motto has become "Your academic career is a marathon, not a sprint." The most important thing is to stay in the race. However, you don't have to proceed full steam ahead all the time. It is OK to stop, slow down, cut back or change priorities, but stay in the game! In the end, at the finish line, you most likely will be toe to toe with your male colleagues. In fact, your energy level may even be greater as a result of your diverse experiences.

However, you can't expect to do it all. Choices must be made. My choice was to hire help at home. My housekeeper cooked dinner (with my recipes), as I had cherished the family dinners during my childhood. She also often drove my carpool. However, I was at the baseball and basketball games, at school programs, at conferences, at Halloween parades, and I often was the chaperone on school trips. I did Suzuki violin with my older son, Richard, and spent Sunday afternoons at his youth symphony rehearsals. I made out the grocery lists, and my husband did the shopping. I limited my travel when my children were young and turned down or elected not to go to many national and international meetings. Did it cost me? Probably, as such meetings are where the connections are made and where name recognition is gained. I did, however, choose to sit on several NIH study sections. The ability to write and receive grants is the life blood of a laboratory investigator. Without grants, we cannot hire personnel or perform the laboratory investigations that will support our academic promotion and progress. Serving on these study sections turned out to be an invaluable experience. Not only did I see the latest science and learn what made an excellent grant, but I also met the experts in my field and in other related disciplines. These individuals learned to respect me as a result of my grant reviews and discussions, and that in turn opened up numerous opportunities for me. It also helped my grant writing skills tremendously, which added to my success in obtaining peer-reviewed funding.

Making time for oneself is often difficult but nonetheless critical for one's mental and physical health. For me, exercise was and still is a very important outlet, and I made it a priority to get to my aerobics class at least three days a week. This was tough, as there was always one more thing to do at work, but I made myself get up and leave. Going to a timed class helped because I couldn't be late. Later I even became certified to teach aerobics and weight training. Besides being incredible fun and giving me a totally different identity, this activity greatly helped my public speaking skills, my confidence in front of an audience, and my ability to think on my feet and respond to questions. I loved the look on people's faces when I told them what my "day job" was! In addition, exercising allowed me to enjoy cookies a few times a week (I am a cookie and chocolate lover but don't care much for cakes).

Another of my favorite sayings is "It's garbage in and garbage out." Forget the fad diets. Count calories and eat what you want. And this is exactly the philosophy I practiced when my younger son decided in fifth grade that he was tired of being fat. It was interfering with his success as a baseball player, as he couldn't run fast. Together we planned meals on the basis of calories. I showed him how to read labels, keep a food diary and count calories during the week. We cheated a little on weekends so that he had something to look forward to and could stay on the program. I showed him how to gauge exercise calorie output so that he could adjust his diet according to his daily activities. He lost 20 pounds over six months and has never slipped back. I am so proud of him for this. Because of his arm and his ability to cover the territory, he was the starting center fielder on his high school baseball team and was later recruited to Johns Hopkins to play.

An important lesson that I learned from my father is that you must know the rules of the game and what you will be judged on. In academic medicine, what counts for promotion are papers and grants. Rarely are you rewarded for being a good teacher or mentor. That doesn't mean you shouldn't do these things. You should! But understand that such activities will gain you few points, so do not neglect publishing and obtaining peer-reviewed funding. Don't think that being liked, being affable and taking extra clinic duty or extra journal clubs will help you get promoted or receive tenure. When the door is closed, the committee will judge you by the rules of engagement.

I have learned to make choices, to listen to my own internal voice and to follow my heart. I have become better at filtering out the snide remarks and criticisms that one encounters, particularly as a woman with a leadership role in a male-dominated occupation. It is imperative to believe in yourself. Others may feel that you are too quiet, too vocal, too petite, not qualified, too young, too old, without experience. What is important, however, is what *you* believe and know to be true about yourself. Look in the mirror and be honest.

What I have also come to learn is that my choice to be a working mother and my husband's help, respect, and support have greatly influenced not only how I conduct myself but also the attitudes of my two sons toward women. They have seen the satisfaction and pride that I derive from my work. They respect women and recognize the importance of a woman's having an independent identity aside from wife and mother. In my opinion, this is a very powerful way to change attitudes. I have learned to lead by example, to lead from the heart, and, most important, to listen to those I lead, allowing them to have a voice in decisions that affect them. I was fortunate to have three superb mentors, all of them male. But I am convinced that without the encouragement and support of my husband, Leonard, I would not be where I am today. He believed in my abilities, pushed me to pursue my dreams and cheered every one of my endeavors. He has been my biggest fan and gave me the confidence that I needed. To young women physicians and scientists, I would say that forging a successful career in this field is a struggle that requires hard work, determination, focus, and juggling priorities, but the rewards are rich and definitely worth the investment of time, energy and tears.

Ritsuko Komaki, M.D.

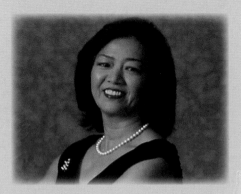

Professor of Radiation Oncology
The Gloria Lupton Tennison Distinguished
Professorship in Lung Cancer

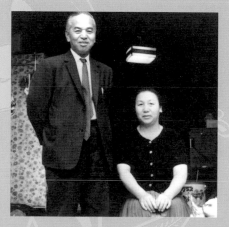

Ritsuko's father Isao Yeda and mother Ykeiko Yeda are shown at home in a suburb of Hiroshima City, Japan, in 1965.

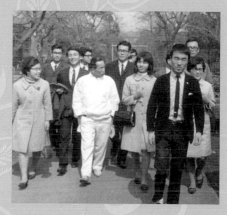

As a medical student at Hiroshima University, Ritsuko (front row, third from left) went with other students to visit basic science departments.

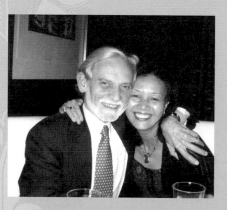

Husband Jim Cox, M.D., was on hand in 2006 when Ritsuko received the award of The Society in Tribute to Marie Skolodowska-Curie in Warsaw, Poland.

y decision to become a cancer researcher and physician was triggered by events early in my life. When Ms. Sadako Sasaki, one of my elementary school friends in Hiroshima, died of acute granulocytic leukemia at the age of 11 after having been exposed to atomic bomb radiation in infancy, I knew that I wanted to be a leukemia researcher or physician so that in the future I would be able to help those with illnesses like hers. Today, I am a professor of radiation oncology at M. D. Anderson Cancer Center and treat patients with thoracic malignancies. My interests include clinical trials, multidisciplinary treatment, normal tissue toxicities and translational research.

Growing up, my role model was Marie Sklodowska-Curie, a respected scientist and the first woman to receive two Nobel prizes: one (together with her husband Pierre) for Physics in 1903, based on their work on natural radioactivity, earlier discovered by Antoine Henri Becquerel, with whom they shared that prize; and the second for Chemistry in 1911, based on the identification and production of metallic radium and the description of the transmutation of one element into another. I find Madame Curie's story inspiring and have read her biography so many times that I know part of her life story from memory. She was a scientist, a wife and the mother of two daughters. Her husband Pierre, who shared his work (and the Nobel Prize in Physics) with his wife, had died in an accident when their daughters were still young. In 1904, Pierre had been given a chair in the School of Physics at the Sorbonne and promised a new laboratory. The laboratory was not forthcoming, however. Then, tragedy struck on April 19, 1906, on a rainy Paris street when Pierre was run over and killed by a horse-drawn carriage while walking from his laboratory.

Marie Curie's background in Poland, where she grew up, was fascinating to me. During the Russian occupation of Poland, Polish children were forced to read their textbooks in Russian in front of Russian soldiers who came to the schools to observe the students' performance under Russian rule. Marie was usually picked by her teachers to read textbooks in Russian since she was the best student in her class and her school. I am certain that her desire to be free from this oppressive environment and her enthusiasm to expand her scientific knowledge motivated her to escape from Poland to France in order to successfully continue her education and become a leader in the scientific community.

Her older sister was already in Paris to study, and this no doubt helped Marie follow in her sister's footsteps. Since Marie's father was a teacher, she had always had an interest in education. I was fascinated reading about her persistence as she discovered polonium while seeking the cause of radioactivity in large amounts of pitchblende ore. Even after her husband's sudden and unexpected death, her passion to investigate radioactivity based on the theory she and Pierre had developed never weakened, and her persistence to forge ahead was never destroyed.

During my childhood in Hiroshima, I had heard many terrible stories of deaths related to radiation from the atomic bomb; these deaths were due to the acute or late effects of the radiation, which included malignancies, psychological depression and suicides. I began to think about who had been responsible for the discovery of radioactivity and radium, about how it originally had been intended for use to alleviate suffering in humans, and about how radiation affects humans. It is ironic that the discovery of radioactive material eventually killed Marie Curie but even more ironic that her persistence to achieve her scientific goals combined with my friend Sadako's death from radiation exposure inspired me to devote my life to becoming a scientist, clinician and educator.

As I was growing up, my parents and their experiences had a great influence on my development and career. My father, Mr. Isao Ueda, was the youngest of 12 children of the family who owned the Sake Brewery on one of the small islands near Hiroshima. My grandfather had died when my father was 10 years old, and his oldest brother had assumed leadership of the family business. When a severe typhoon hit the inland sea, the family-owned ship carrying Sake barrels sunk and left the business and the family bankrupt and without any insurance coverage. Thus, at the age of 13, my father had to go to work delivering Sake bottles for his oldest brother's new small liquor store in Hiroshima so that he could stay in his brother's house. My father decided to get a scholarship to the Hiroshima University School of Education, but this meant that he had to commit to teaching children ages 7 to 12 in a small village for four years after completing his education. The period in that tiny village was the most boring time of his life and he developed a peptic ulcer, but he was nevertheless able to save his money and then pass the entrance examination for admission to Kyoto University, where he majored in economics.

After graduating from Kyoto University, he married my mother in an arranged marriage, went to work in Osaka, a city approximately 250 miles east and north of Hiroshima and the second largest city in Japan (after Tokyo), and began working for Hanshin, one of the most prestigious companies. Then, at 8:15 a.m. on August 6, 1945, the atomic bomb was dropped on Hiroshima. The following day, my father walked into Hiroshima and was exposed to "black rain" containing a high dose of radiation. He lost many members of his family who were exposed to high levels of radiation from the bomb, although some family members exposed to the radiation managed to survive. My father decided to move back to Hiroshima to help his and my mother's families and took a job in the Hiroshima Bank. I recall that every time he was promoted to chief of a different branch of the bank, we had to move to a different city. I had to change school four times while still in elementary school, although I never complained. When we moved to Matsuyama, a small city on Shikoku Island, my teacher there always asked me to read aloud from the textbook in our class. My classmates laughed at me because of my Hiroshima accent, and this made me furious.

My father was always busy and often came home around 2 a.m. As a banker, he had to entertain his customers after 6 p.m. every night. I never saw him other than on Sunday; I always missed him and was puzzled by the Japanese work system. He was the leader of the union and eventually retired at age 55 when he was not promoted to executive member in the Hiroshima Bank. By virtue of his education, he should have been one of the executives, but the other executive members feared his idealism and higher education than theirs. He eventually died of disseminated bladder cancer at age 72, possibly due to his exposure to the atomic bomb radiation and to his tobacco smoking. He smoked one to two packs a day of Peace for at least 40 years. I always feared that he might develop lung cancer, but instead, he developed diabetes, bladder cancer and peripheral vascular disease. My father was a very hard-working man, but he was so disappointed by his first child's (and only son's) incurable illness that it caused him to be very distant from his three daughters, of which I was the middle daughter. Because of my father's remoteness, I always felt that his daughters did not mean much to him, and I wished that I had been born a boy so that I could have fulfilled his desire for a son.

My mother, whose maiden name was Yukiko Obata, was the oldest daughter of a samurai family. Her father (my maternal grandfather, Mr. Kanbei Obata) had graduated from Tokyo University and had once served as a chief officer of the Ministry of Agriculture in Japan. After his retirement, my grandfather had served as a secretary to Mr. Asano, lord of the Hiroshima prefecture. My grandparents had a huge samurai house with several maids and secretaries to serve them. My mother was raised by a babysitter, as my grandmother was too busy visiting temples and shrines to care for her. My grandmother was my grandfather's second wife, after he had lost his first wife to tuberculosis. He had decided to marry my grandmother because she was the strongest woman in town. A striking woman, my grandmother was 6 feet tall, with red hair and fair skin, and everyone said that she had one-eighth Russian blood. Men found her imposing height intimidating, and she had not previously found a husband because men considered her "too tall to marry." For many men, marrying a small cute and very obedient wife was one of the most important marriage criteria in Japan. My mother was extremely proud of her samurai family background (on my grandfather's side) and blamed her marriage to a lower-class person (my father) on the first world war. She spoke about her grandmother, "Chika," who was for her the most elegant and caring person. My mother truly loved me and would demonstrate her affection, for example, by hugging me when I got a good grade in school. I never received such affection from my father or anyone else. By the age of 7, my mother had read almost all of the books in her father's library. Because of his position as secretary of a Lord, he had many books on European and Asian history, and my mother read and memorized all of them.

In later years, when my husband and I took my mother to France and Vienna, she was our guide for information on the European royal family trees. She read many Chinese and Russian history books and all 12 volumes of Pearl Buck's "Big Earth" about China. However, her incredible knowledge of world history did not help to support family members when the atomic bomb destroyed everything. Thus, she wanted her three daughters to become capable women who could support the family in case anything should happen to their spouses. My mother had great pride but was always extremely kind to those less fortunate. She told me to give my extra pencils and notebooks to some of my classmates who were orphaned after the atomic bomb or to those whose fathers had died in the war. For her entire life, my mother loved to cook for us and to compose Haiku (Japanese poems). After my father died and she traveled with us, her knowledge about the histories of Japan and European countries and her ability to compose beautiful Haiku amazed us and others wherever we went. My mother died of stomach cancer at the age of 80. I still miss her very much.

I was born in Amagasaki, a city in the Hyogo prefecture between Osaka and Kobe, while my father, Mr. Isao Ueda, was working in Osaka. I was my parents' third child. My family decided to move back to Hiroshima when I was 4 years old, since they had originally come from that city and since they had to return there to help family members who had survived the bombing. However, after we moved back to Hiroshima, we had to move again many times due to the lack of housing and to my father's promotions in the Hiroshima Bank. I had to change elementary schools four times within six years.

I met my friend Sadako Sasaki in the Nobori-Cho Elementary School when I was 10 years old and in the fifth grade. We were the same age but in different classes in order to compete in running events in the fall athletic meeting. Sadako was very fast, and I had a tough time racing against her. At the age of 2, Sadako had been exposed to radiation from the atomic bomb. She eventually developed shortness of breath due to anemia and was diagnosed with leukemia. She was hospitalized and died of leukemia nine months after her diagnosis. Before she became ill, she had registered to attend Nobori-Cho Junior High School; sadly, she never was able to do that. While Sadako was hospitalized, she attempted to fold 1,000 origami cranes. In Japan, the crane is a symbol of longevity and happiness. It is said that if you can fold 1,000 cranes, you can recover from your illness. After Sadako took her medication, she folded her origami cranes from the wax paper that had wrapped her medication. Sadako wanted to live! However, despite our prayers and our helping her fold her cranes, she passed away. Two years after her death, I became president of the junior high school that she had registered to enter but never gotten to attend. When she died, all the children in the school expressed their sorrow to her brothers and parents.

When I became president of Nobori-Cho Junior High School, I began to communicate more often with Sadako's older brother. He and I started to initiate plans for a memorial statue for her. We decided to go on the streets and gather donations from Hiroshima's citizens, and we also wrote many letters to deans of schools in Japan asking for funding contributions for her memorial. We also engaged a young gentleman, Mr. Kawamoto, to help us get a public educational film-making group to create "Sadako's Story," which became a hit film titled "One Thousand Cranes" and was shown in many movie theaters. Within two years, we had collected enough funding to hire an architect to create an "atomic bomb children's statue" in the center of the Peace Memorial Park in Hiroshima on the site of the hypo-center where the bomb had been dropped.

Sadako's death had a very profound influence on me. Although I was very sad, I also realized that I now had a mission: to make sure that Sadako's death would not be forgotten and to send a message to younger generations that destructive wars that destroy so many lives should never be allowed to happen again. Also, I was very curious about the effects of atomic bomb radiation, since my grandmother had been in Hiroshima when the bomb was dropped. In fact, her house had collapsed due to the suction effects from the bomb. She was trapped underneath her house but was rescued from the ruins and taken outside of the city. In the few months that followed, she experienced every side effect of total-body radiation (e.g., hair loss, severe diarrhea, anorexia and bone marrow suppression). However, she recovered from these effects and lived an almost normal life without developing leukemia or any malignancy. My grandmother died of severe senile dementia and osteoporosis at the age of 72. I was always puzzled by why she did not develop leukemia as Sadako had. Now I have a much better understanding of this, as I have learned about the higher susceptibility to carcinogens in the dividing cells of younger individuals.

I decided to attend medical school, but my parents wanted me to stay in Hiroshima, since it would take six years to graduate and they did not want me separated from them for that long. Thus, I entered Hiroshima University School of Medicine. While I was a medical student, I volunteered during summer vacations to perform physical examinations of people who had been exposed to atomic bomb radiation at the Atomic Bomb Casualty Commission (ABCC), now called the Radiation Effect Research Foundation (RERF). While working at the RERF, I met Dr. Awa, one of the world's leading experts on the chromosome abnormality caused by radiation, and became very interested in hematology and chromosome abnormalities. I also met Dr. Bloom, a hematologist, Dr. Bell, a thyroid specialist, and Dr. Robert, a cardiologist who was checking cardiac effects in humans exposed to atomic bomb radiation. At the RERF in Hiroshima, I had a wonderful opportunity to meet with great scientists and clinicians who were interested in radiation effects on humans.

Then, when I graduated from Hiroshima University School of Medicine, all the interns and medical students at our Hiroshima University Hospital as well as all other university hospitals decided to go on strike. We were protesting to have the government pay for the internships and improve the medical system and the medical school curricula at the University Hospitals. We had to go outside the University Hospitals to get postgraduate education by ourselves. I went back to the RERF in Hiroshima and worked for a year, during which time I married Dr. Senichiro Komaki, a diagnostic radiologist from Kyushu University working at the RERF. We came to the United States to continue our postgraduate education at the Medical College of Wisconsin (MCW) in Milwaukee. By order of his professor, my husband had to go back to Kyushu University, which led to our divorce, since I wanted to continue my residency program in Milwaukee. He subsequently remarried and died of adenocarcinoma of the lung several years ago.

I started my internship at St. Mary's Hospital in Milwaukee, where I met Dr. Guenninger, who had a double specialty: internal medicine and radiation oncology. He was well respected by the surgeons and medical oncologists with whom I was working. I started to think about radiation oncology as a specialty, but because of my original interest in hematology-oncology, I began work at the Wood VA Hospital in Milwaukee as a hematology-oncology fellow. However, the results in patients treated by chemotherapy around that time were not great. Most of the time I had to deal with anemic patients at the VA Hospital. However, when I began seeing some patients whose early laryngeal cancer or Hodgkin disease was cured by radiotherapy, I decided to enter a radiation oncology residency program at MCW in 1974. With my background having come from Hiroshima, radiation oncology was a fascinating area for me.

After I went back to MCW, I focused on a multidisciplinary treatment approach for cancer patients and learned much from the physicians and researchers I met during my residency there: about surgical oncology from Dr. William Donagen; gynecologic oncology from Dr. Richard Mattingly;

pathology from Dr. Lawry Clowry; pediatric oncology from Drs. Larry Kun and Donald Pinkel; lung, head and neck, genitourinary cancer, and lymphoma from Drs. James D. Cox, Roger Byhardt, and Donald Eisert; breast and brachytherapy from J. Frank Wilson; and physics from Dr. Michael Gillin. I was the first and only resident when I started the residency program at MCW under the new department chairman, Dr. James D. Cox. I was well taught by famous radiation oncologists who were all interested in a multidisciplinary approach. When I first came to M. D. Anderson Hospital and Tumor Institute (as it was then called) as an observer for three months in 1980, Dr. Gilbert H. Fletcher was still chairman of the Department of Radiation Oncology.

I wanted to be an expert in gynecologic oncology and came to follow Dr. Fletcher's clinic. His knowledge in head and neck and gynecologic oncology was truly impressive. Again, I met so many great radiation oncologists (Drs. Gilbert Fletcher, David Hussey, Nora Tapley, Eleanor Montague, Lillian Fuller, Luis Delclos, Thomas Berkley, Robert Lindberg, and Rodney Withers) and gynecologic and head and neck oncologists here at M. D. Anderson.

At that time, I never imagined working at such a prestigious institution as M. D. Anderson, but now I have been here almost 20 years. I completed my radiation oncology residency program at MCW in 1979 and then did my fellowship for nine months at MCW and observed for three months at M. D. Anderson in 1980. I stayed at MCW and became an associate professor of radiation oncology. My specialty was gynecologic oncology, and my interests were in predictors of gynecologic malignancies, including histologic grading, ploidy, DNA index, anemia and other factors. At MCW, I taught medical students during summers, and many of them are now professors of radiation oncology there, including Beth Erickson, Colleen Lawton and Chris Shultz. Because of Dr. Eric Hall's reputation working with radiation effects on humans and also because of persistent recruitment by Dr. Chu Chang, one of the kindest physicians we met in New York City, Dr. James D. Cox accepted a position as chairman of the Radiation Oncology department at Columbia Presbyterian Medical Center in 1985. This new department was created 40 years after the last department, Anesthesiology, had been created. Jim and I had married in 1980, and so I tagged along on this new endeavor.

At Columbia Presbyterian Medical Center, I obtained a position as a clinical chief and associate professor of radiation oncology and treated many patients with breast, gynecologic and lung cancers. I introduced conservative surgery followed by radiotherapy for early breast cancer, which was not routine there at that time. Dr. Frank Gump was one of the open-minded breast cancer surgeons there and became very collaborative with Dr. James D. Cox and me.

Jim Cox and I worked hard to make the Radiation Oncology department at Columbia Presbyterian better. We met great people there, but clinical trials and studies were very difficult to conduct. We decided to move to M. D. Anderson Cancer Center when Jim was offered a position there as vice president of patient care and physician-in-chief in 1988. Dr. Lester Peters, the division head of Radiation Oncology at that time, recruited me as a section chief of Thoracic Radiation Oncology and an associate professor of radiation oncology. I have learned so much about radiation oncology here at M. D. Anderson — about radiation pneumonitis from Dr. Elizabeth Travis, radiation time/fractionation of head and neck cancer from Drs. Lester Peters and Kian Ang, and translational research from Dr. Luka Milas.

Highlights in my professional life include becoming president of the Japan-U.S. Cancer Therapy Symposium (JUCTS) in 1999, president of the American Association for Women Radiologists (AAWR) in 2001, and president of the American Radium Society in 2007-2008; receiving a Texas Women Business Award in 2005, the Marie Sklodowska-Curie Award in 2005, and an award from The Society in Tribute to Maria Sklodowska-Curie in Warsaw, Poland, in 2006. I wish that my mother had been with us when I received the Marie Curie Award. She would have been so proud of me and would have hugged me, saying, " Ri-chan (my nick name), you have done a great job!"

One more highlight for me, along with Jim Cox and others, was opening the M. D. Anderson Proton Therapy Center in May 2006. Proton treatment has been one of our dreams to reduce side effects to normal tissue, especially in children. After being raised in Hiroshima, I have always felt that radiation is a double-edged sword, as Eric Hall said. If a low dose of radiation is scattered over the body, the incidence of a second malignancy will increase, especially among children or long-term cancer survivors. On the other hand, proton treatment with active scanning to remove neutrons will deliver a very sharp beam edge without scattering the radiation, thus reducing the chance of second malignancies.

In my personal life, a major highlight was my marriage to Jim Cox, who has been my mentor, friend, advisor, supporter and a wonderful husband. My hobbies are traveling, visiting gardens (especially Japanese gardens), and orchid and other flower arrangements. Also, I love to talk to children about my friend Sadako and about how to make origami cranes. And of course, I would like to let them know how terrible nuclear (and any other) war is and why it must be prevented.

There have been many sad memories in my life, including my brother's illness, Sadako's death, my parents' and my patients' deaths due to cancer, and Valerie Cox's death due to an automobile accident when she was 18 years old. Whenever I faced those tragedies, Marie Curie's words encouraged me. As she said, "Life is not easy for anybody. But what of that? We must have our perseverance and above all, confidence in ourselves. We must believe that we are gifted for something and this must be attained."... "Nothing in life is to be feared. It is only to be understood," and " One never notices what has been done; one can only see what remains to be done."

Finally, I thank all great clinicians, managers, nurses, therapists, physicists, dosimetrists and dietitians who care for patients, and scientists and educators who take care of trainees and fellows at M. D. Anderson. I will continue to learn about science, care for patients, teach others and give messages from Sadako, Marie Curie, my mother and my patients, who all still live in my mind and always will.

Margaret L. Kripke, Ph.D.

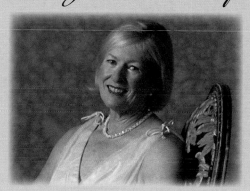

Special Advisor to the Provost
Professor of Immunology
Vivian L. Smith Distinguished Chair in Immunology, Emerita

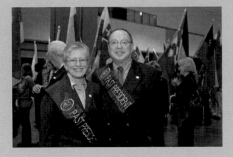

Margaret and husband Isaiah (Josh) Fidler, D.V.M., Ph.D., are the only married couple to have served as presidents of the American Association for Cancer Research since the organization was founded in 1907.

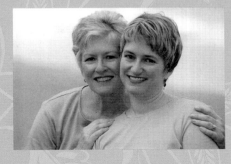

In 2002, Margaret and horse Charleston competed in a three-day Texas cross country course.

(Photo by Jim Stoner Photography)

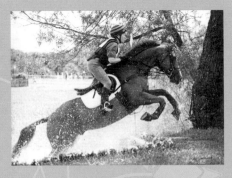

Daughter Katherine Kripke helped Margaret celebrate her 60th birthday at Lake Tahoe in 2003.

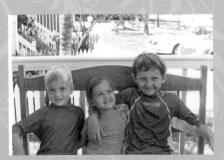

Favorite photo subjects for Margaret and Josh are their grandchildren, from left, Evan, 7, Eden, 3, and Jake, 9.

t seems to me that I have always loved natural science, particularly biology. I have no doubt that this proclivity came, in large measure, from my father, who was an amateur naturalist and a great gardener. Although my parents were products of the Great Depression and had little formal education, they were interested in learning and made the effort to take an occasional night class at a junior college in a nearby town. Dinner conversations often centered around Dad's classes in anthropology and archeology. I knew about Darwin's theory of natural selection and survival of the fittest before I went to high school, and I had heard about Margaret Mead's and Ruth Benedict's studies of other cultures long before I took anthropology in college. Because there were no boys in the family, I became the surrogate son and gardened and fished with my father, while my older sister took up more traditional female activities. I suppose this formed the basis for my assumption that girls need not be limited to traditional roles and for my expectation that I could do whatever I wanted professionally.

From kindergarten to college, I lived in a small town in an agricultural region of northern California. I was always a good student; I read lots of books, took all the elective courses my school had to offer, played classical piano, and was strongly encouraged by my parents to do more. In retrospect, it is clear that they were trying to keep me out of trouble by keeping me as busy as possible! Since this was the immediate post-Sputnik era, science was pushed strongly in schools. In my junior year of high school, I was selected to attend a summer program for potential scientists at Santa Clara University, sponsored by the National Science Foundation. Predictably, I gravitated toward the biology projects and loved every minute of the experience. As a senior in high school, I was a cheerleader and a valedictorian and thought about writing a book titled "I was a teenage spinster," owing to the fact that several of my friends were married in or shortly after high school. I knew, however, that this was not my goal in life; I was college-bound and determined to see more of the world than my immediate environs. Finances and a scholarship conspired to keep me close to home, however. In 1961, I headed off to the University of California at Berkeley to study zoology, becoming the first member of my family to attend a major university.

My thoughts of a career in those days didn't extend beyond a vague hope that I might someday go to medical school. However, the transition from being first in my small class to being one among thousands of bright kids in classes larger than my entire high school took its toll on my grades. I did well in biological sciences and fine arts but poorly in social and physical sciences. It took me the first two years just to figure out how to study. Meanwhile, there were distractions — beer, bridge and boys (of course) — and there were also political issues — the Free Speech Movement, Civil Rights and later, the Vietnam War, the sexual revolution and gay rights. I did my share of marching and sitting in, but in the end, my heart still belonged to biology. Although it wasn't apparent to me at the time, I learned some things about leadership during those years. My role models were the leader of the Free Speech Movement, a Berkeley student named Mario Savio, the Reverend Martin Luther King and President John F. Kennedy. (And yes, I remember exactly where I was when the president was assassinated.) Charisma, passion and an inspiring message seemed to be the common characteristics of these successful leaders.

Toward the end of my undergraduate years, it was clear I wasn't going to medical school. In those days, only the select few at the top of their class could get in, and for women, this was doubly true. Unlike today, when women make up around 50 percent of medical school classes, in the mid-1960s women were still an anomaly in this setting and not particularly welcome additions. Besides, there was the cost issue. After my parents had sacrificed to send me to college, I wouldn't think of asking them to continue to support me beyond graduation. So while I was agonizing over what on earth I was going to do with a degree in zoology, a miracle happened. The summer before my senior year, I received an invitation from my professors in bacteriology to come and talk to them about my career plans, since I had done well in their course. This occurred because there was concern at Berkeley that undergraduate students were not receiving enough attention from the faculty. In addition, generous funding was available for student stipends in all areas of science, again because of the post-Sputnik push to upgrade science in America. These fortuitous circumstances were responsible for my scientific career. I was quickly rechanneled into an undergraduate major in bacteriology and immunology and was admitted to graduate school (with a stipend), in spite of my less than stellar academic record.

In graduate school, I quickly found my niche in the research lab. My parents diplomatically suppressed their concerns that I was graduating from college without either a husband or a job and that I was going to remain a student for another few years. They remained supportive, however, and helped out with expenses when needed. As a second-year graduate student, I married an assistant professor of mathematics and, in doing so, improved my lifestyle and my bridge game as well as my understanding of statistics. Shortly thereafter, my thesis advisor (one of the bacteriology professors who had rescued me), emigrated to Israel to become chair of the Department of Immunology at the Hebrew University-Hadassah Medical School in Jerusalem. This afforded me the opportunity to explore one of my life's goals, which was to see more of the world. I convinced my husband to take a sabbatical and finish a book he was writing, and, after a crash course in Hebrew, we went off to Israel.

This was a phenomenal learning experience for me, little of which had to do with science. I learned as much about my own country as I did about my host country. Living in a Jewish state taught me a lot about the significance of separation of church and state. Living in a country with socialized medicine illustrated both the advantages and limitations of our own medical system. Similarly, observing a political system that involved a coalition government improved my understanding of the pros and cons of our two-party system. Most of all, it made me appreciate how many things we take for granted in the United States that simply are not available in other parts of the world. I concluded that every American teenager should spend a year living in another country in order to develop an appreciation of the privileges they enjoy simply by being born in the United States.

Somehow in the two years we were in Jerusalem, I managed to complete my thesis research and become pregnant. My daughter Katharine was born in Hadassah Hospital two months before we were to return to the United States. By then, I had finished my lab work (the six-day work week helped a lot) and was finishing writing my thesis. It seemed like a convenient time to have a baby since there would be a gap between completing my thesis and starting postdoctoral work. So I returned from Israel with a Ph.D. and a new baby.

Since it had been my choice to go to Israel, it was my husband's choice where we went next. While in Israel, he had decided to leave mathematics and become a neurophysiologist, so he began seeking training opportunities in that field. For three months after we returned to the States, we drove cross country, visiting the two sets of grandparents, first in New York and then in California. Along the way, we visited some potential labs for my husband and eventually ended up at Ohio State University in Columbus, where he began to work and apply for fellowships to support his retraining. Needless, to say, I needed a job quickly and was fortunate to find a postdoctoral position with a professor of microbiology and immunology who had recently joined the faculty.

During that period, I suffered my first professional disappointment and my first encounter with gender discrimination. My thesis research, which I, of course, thought was brilliant, was rejected for publication by the *Journal of the National Cancer Institute*. I was devastated and ready to give up my research career, believing I had failed as a scientist. Once again, I was rescued by my thesis advisor, who patiently explained that this was not the end of my career and that I needed to address the criticisms of the reviewers and resubmit the paper to another journal whose editor was more sympathetic to the issue of immune surveillance. He was right, of course. The paper was accepted without revision and published in the *International Journal of Cancer*. The discrimination issue, however, did not have as satisfying an outcome. During my job search, I was asked to interview with a professor in the medical school. After talking with me for a while, he apologized that he didn't really have a position open at the moment, remarking that it was a shame that his two postdocs (both male) had just hired a technician (female), since otherwise, I would have been perfect for that job. While I was digesting this comment, he asked me if I had any possibilities for a job elsewhere, and I replied truthfully that I did although the position didn't pay very well, so I had not accepted it yet. At that point, he proceeded to assure me that there should be no problem since I was married and my husband could support me. Rather than try to explain that my husband was jobless at the moment and I had an extra mouth to feed as well as child care expenses to pay, I thanked him for his time and left. I could have explained or complained then or later, but I felt it was futile since there seemed to be no common ground between our points of view. Today, I would probably behave differently, but at the time, it was probably a wise choice to walk away, avoid burning bridges and concentrate on other, more immediate battles, like getting a job.

My postdoctoral period was again a great learning experience. This time I learned more science and broadened my perspective considerably. I also learned something about what it was like to be a Black professional in America, since my professor was African-American. Against that backdrop, gender discrimination seemed somehow less important. Because I had been a Civil Rights sympathizer, if not an activist, in my Berkeley days, we had much to talk about. Toward the end of my second year, I received an unsolicited invitation to interview for a position in the Department of Pathology at the University of Utah in Salt Lake City. The job was a non-tenure-track research faculty position that involved running a large National Cancer Institute (NCI) research contract dealing with immune suppression and skin cancer. When I read the job description, I knew it was the perfect project for me. Immune surveillance and cancer was the subject of my thesis research, and I felt that I knew as much about the subject as anyone else in the country. Even though my postdoctoral mentor had recently become a department chair and had offered me a tenure-track faculty position in his department, I responded immediately to the invitation from the University of Utah and arranged for both my husband and me to go for interviews.

It was indeed the perfect project for me, and a wonderful environment. The only negatives were that the position was non-tenure track and that there was no faculty position available for my husband. I somehow had the foresight to ask about the possibility of my receiving a tenure-track position. In response, I was asked why I felt I needed one. My answer was that I had been offered one elsewhere and that it would look much better on my resume if I went elsewhere in the future. The department chair went back to the dean with my request, and it was granted, partly because I was a perfect fit for the job and they needed me to run the project but mostly because there were so few women on the medical school faculty that it was advantageous for the school. This time, and in all my subsequent appointments, the gender issue actually worked in my favor. As predicted, my work went exceptionally well, and I made discoveries that formed the basis of my lifelong scientific career.

I very quickly began to develop national recognition. I can identify three factors that helped me in this regard. The first was my discovery of the unusual immunologic properties of ultraviolet light-induced skin cancers, which was published in the *Journal of the National Cancer Institute*. I actually received a personal letter from the editor thanking me for submitting my work there; this was especially heartwarming in light of my rejection of a few years earlier. Second, I had wonderful mentors. The chair of my department taught me a great deal about science, administration and focus; another pathology colleague and director of the research contract taught me organizational skills and transplantation immunology; and a professor of biology and a consultant on the contract taught me photobiology and introduced me to the American Society for Photobiology. Years later, I served as president of this society and received both its Research and Lifetime Achievement awards. All of these colleagues served as critics, mentors and advocates for my work and career. Third, I developed a productive working relationship with the sponsors of our research contract at the NCI, which gained me additional external recognition and another source of career support and advocacy within the granting agency.

Meanwhile, my husband had managed to carve a niche for himself by using his talents as a teacher and supporting part of his salary from a research grant. Although we both loved our work and were happy in Salt Lake City, our marriage did not survive. Having grown up with a serious case of the "Cinderella Complex," I was uncomfortable in the role of primary family professional. My expectation that my successful assistant professor of mathematics would simply take care of me the way Prince Charming took care of Cinderella had not materialized, and I was resentful. I can only surmise that the fact that I was sought after and successful academically caused similar resentments on his side. In spite of my determination to make things work, fate intervened. I was invited to speak at a Science Writers' meeting in Florida, sponsored by the American Cancer Society, where I was dazzled by another participant, a flamboyant scientist named Josh Fidler. I came home from the meeting with the sad realization that my marriage was not going to work and that I needed to get on with my life and career. My husband and I parted ways with much pain and regret, particularly for Katharine, who was then just 4, and I became a single, working mother.

Apparently the dazzling was mutual, because Josh made a trip to Salt

Lake City to see me shortly thereafter. We decided to explore places to go to be together. We were extremely fortunate during the next year to be invited, independent of each other, to look at laboratory director positions at the newly created NCI-Frederick Cancer Research Center in Maryland. Although Josh was offered a position in Salt Lake City, it was too far from his children, who were then 6 and 8 and living in Philadelphia. The positions in Frederick seemed like a reasonable option, even though Josh gave up a tenured faculty position at the University of Pennsylvania to go there and even though there was a high level of uncertainty that the center would succeed. In 1975, we went to Frederick and began the first of our 32 years of marriage.

The Frederick years were both difficult and wonderful. Work was terrifically successful for both of us. We lived in a small town where Katharine could walk to school and I could run home at a moment's notice. After a few years, my mother joined us in Frederick, which enabled me to be more active in attending scientific meetings, and my career thrived. The director of the research program taught me a great deal and was a great advocate for my career. He gave me opportunities for leadership that were invaluable. Since I was new at the leadership game, I made many mistakes and suffered the consequences. This was a critical, though painful, period of growth in my career as a leader. I had to learn how to deal with difficult people, how to fire underperformers, how to listen, how to give honest feedback and how to accept disappointments. I also learned that being authentic is essential for successful leadership. As with all good things, this era also came to an end. There were leadership changes at the NCI that suggested our idyllic existence was likely to change. Also, we were facing the prospect of three children going to college and needed a more secure working environment than the center could offer.

Once again, we were phenomenally lucky in our professional lives. Josh and I previously had both turned down opportunities to look at other positions because we were so comfortable personally and professionally in Frederick. However, when things began to change, I insisted that we needed to look elsewhere. Since Josh had been approached about positions at M. D. Anderson Cancer Center several times in recent years, he took the initiative to inquire whether there were appropriate openings for us there. Over the next six months, department chair positions and start-up packages materialized for both of us, and the opportunities and the institution were so attractive to us that we never looked anywhere else. Again, I believe the gender issue played in my favor. I was the first female chair of an academic department at M. D. Anderson, and again, life was both satisfying and challenging professionally. During the ensuing years, I garnered support and recognition for my research, trained students and fellows, and built a fledgling

Department of Immunology from scratch. Also in that time, Josh and I became the first and, to date, only couple to have both been elected president of the American Association for Cancer Research.

I was given many opportunities for leadership and participation at the institutional level, which helped me succeed in a highly male-dominated environment. In recounting my mentors, all of whom have been male, I cannot fail to acknowledge my husband, who has been my strongest supporter, fiercest protector and most astute political advisor. He has also allowed me to develop as a leader, even though sometimes it has created hardships for him professionally and socially.

After 15 years as a department chair, I began to feel that I and the department needed a change. I was not learning anything new administratively, my science and students were suffering from lack of attention, and my department needed greater strength in basic and translational immunology than I could provide. I therefore informed my supervisor that I would be stepping down within the next two years, either to return to my laboratory or to pursue other administrative opportunities.

To help clarify my next course of action, I applied for an executive leadership development course designed specifically for women in academic medicine (The Executive Leadership in Academic Medicine Program). During that year-long curriculum, I again learned a great deal about leadership, my personal style, and my strengths and weaknesses as a leader. In the end, it was clear that I was ready to give up my successful research career, although reluctantly, to take on new leadership challenges at a higher level. Fortunately, timing was on my side because a new president had just been appointed. The institutional restructuring that took place shortly thereafter provided the chance for me to advance to a new leadership role. I am most grateful for the opportunities to grow and learn that resulted from my successive roles as Vice President, Senior Vice President, and eventually, Executive Vice President for Academic Programs. I am also appreciative to those who helped facilitate my appointment by President Bush as a member of the President's Cancer Panel, which reports to the White House on issues of concern in our nation's cancer program.

It is not possible for me to recount all the lessons I learned in these roles or to thank all those who helped me. My goals in assuming this leadership role were to bring a new level of transparency and clear criteria for success in our academic enterprise, to help create a more supportive environment for women, to develop a culture of leadership and accountability, and to help improve the quality of research and education in the institution. I will leave it to others to judge the outcomes. However, participating in our faculty leadership development course over the past few years motivates me to end by articulating my own leadership principles.

First, always tell the truth. Consistency is necessary for gaining trust, and besides, it's easier to remember what you said. Second, always be accountable for your actions and take responsibility for your decisions. Third, give people as much information as they need, or at least as much as you can. If you don't, they will make up stories about what is going on. Fourth, strive for excellence, and make decisions based on this guiding principle. Fifth, reward the behavior that you want. Never punish success and never reward bad behavior. There are two other principles that I have used throughout my personal and professional life. One came from my mother, who told me never to put anything in writing that I wouldn't want to see on the front page of the newspaper. This is still good advice, particularly in these days of instant electronic communication. The second principle came from a high school teacher, who said her mother told her to always leave the party while you're still having a good time. I have tried to follow this advice when changing career directions, and it is the main reason that I have recently stepped down from my position as Executive Vice President and am continuing to work only part time. I am looking forward to a more relaxed existence than I have had for the past nine years — one that includes more time to ride my horse, garden, cook, travel and play with the grandchildren. So far, I am not lacking for things to do!

Razelle Kurzrock, M.D.

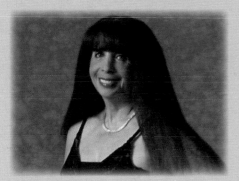

**Professor and Chair of Investigational
Cancer Therapeutics
Anderson Clinical Faculty Chair for
Cancer Treatment and Research**

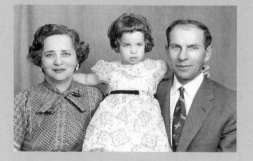

Razelle was 4 in this picture with mother Matilda and father David Kurzrock at home in Toronto, Canada.

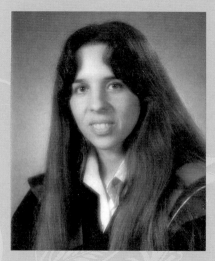

Razelle received her medical degree at age 22 from the University of Toronto in 1978.

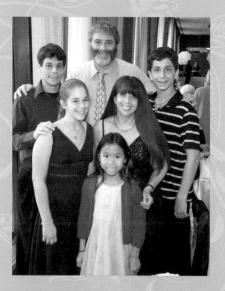

Husband Philip Cohen, M.D., and Razelle with their children, from left, Benjamin, 18; Rena, 12; Tali, 9, and Jonathan, 15, in 2007.

(Mark Katz Photography)

was practically born wanting to be a scientist. I have known that I wanted to be a research scientist and to discover things since I was 6 years old, and this decision was reinforced with the death of my mother from rheumatic heart disease when I was 12. Several specific incidents during my childhood enforced that career decision and showed that I was fairly entrenched in the love of science at a very early age. For example, I remember in the second grade hiding my science book under the table and reading it while other classes were in progress. Unfortunately, I was "discovered," which led to my nickname (mostly by the boys in my class) of "the scientist." Given that I was a somewhat overweight, nerdy child to begin with, being made fun of was painful, but, like all the difficult experiences that could have turned me away from a future in science, it did not deter me from sticking to my early career choice. In the fourth grade, the principal took me aside, along with several other kids in the class, and told us that we were going to be placed into a combined fifth and sixth grade class, so that we would effectively skip a year of elementary school. The teacher of this combined class was excellent and probably was my most influential teacher, but she did one thing that angered me at the time and stuck with me for years. Everyone in the class was assigned the task of writing a biography of a well-known person, and everyone in the class got to choose whom they wrote about — except for me. Instead of letting me choose, my teacher told me that I had to write my assignment on Madame Curie. I was insulted and felt that she didn't think highly enough of me to allow me to make my own choice. It wasn't until years later, when I was in college, that I realized that what I had taken to be an insult years before was actually my teacher's attempt to provide me with an early role model of a woman in science. Since Madame Curie was one of the few scientists to have been awarded two Nobel prizes, it is now clear to me that my teacher wanted Madame Curie's story to inspire me.

Later, as a young adult, one of my earliest and most important choices was my decision to come to M. D. Anderson Cancer Center after leaving Canada and completing my residency in internal medicine at Tulane University. I had been looking for fellowships in oncology and had wanted to find one in a place that was involved in first-in-human studies. I wanted to leave Canada because, although the research in basic science there was innovative and top drawer, the clinical research tended to be conservative and to confirm results from the more advanced clinical studies being done in the United States. The wisdom of my decision to come to M. D. Anderson was reinforced soon after I arrived here, during a conference on bone marrow transplants. At this meeting, one of the faculty members opined that M. D. Anderson should not become involved in carrying out a particular transplant technique, since the leader in that field was in Seattle and this technique was not being performed there. At that point, the moderator of the conference, a scientist of considerable stature, became very agitated and made it clear to the faculty member that M. D. Anderson was *a leader* at the forefront of innovative science and medicine rather than a follower and, indeed, that followers (such as he) did not belong here. Doing pioneering work, I realized, was the predominant value at M. D. Anderson and was just what I had sought — a place that was a leader in scientific discovery. Thus, I knew that I had made the correct decision to come to M. D. Anderson, the unpleasantness of the conference exchange notwithstanding.

If there is one characteristic needed by women to enable them to succeed in medicine and science, it is a dogged persistence to stick by their choices no matter what roadblocks are put in their way. Along my career path, I encountered pivotal incidents and turning points. At some of these junctures, it would have undoubtedly been easier to abandon my goal, but I was resolute, and because my goal had been a focal point of my life for so many years, I persisted. So many of these obstacles or difficulties center around marriage and having children, blending schedules, coordinating career paths, and nurturing one's own career; thus, women in science have to be stubbornly persistent along the way.

Marriage and children present their own particular challenges. These are partially due to the conflicting life plans of the parties involved and also to the amount of time and energy that is required to have a successful career in academics. Often the sheer amount of time and energy that must be devoted to patient care, research and training is distinctly at odds with maintaining a well-balanced family life. The Myth of Sisyphus is probably an excellent metaphor for the struggle of women dedicated to an academic career to stay on track. Like the boulder rolling back down the hill after it is pushed (with great effort) to the top, many life events occur that sometimes call into question whether one actually *can* do it all — have a demanding career, a husband with his own career and life choices, and children with lives to be managed and coordinated. There were many times in my life during the course of forging my successful career that I had to just stick to it, no matter what. But there is no such thing as a free lunch, and being resolute carries its own set of emotional prices. Women who go into science and who want to succeed must be prepared to face many obstacles, sometimes placed there by the very people to whom they are closest.

Women in medicine face unique challenges. Women don't, for the most part, have the natural support system that men have; they often do not have role models. Whereas men are generally appointed to the biggest leadership roles based upon their *potential,* women have to reach their potential before they become leaders in their field. Also, those men who are mentored by other men have a great foot up on the ladder of success. Mentors have a vested interest in the success of the people they choose to mentor. So, if the acolytes succeed, it reflects positively upon the mentor who selected them out of the professional crowd. Children and husbands also are frequently impediments to women in this field. Because women are often very attached to the children and go through pregnancies (and not always easy ones at that), they have an additional gradient, practical and emotional, that must be fit into their careers and squared away. Tradition has it that the husband's career has primacy, whereas it is assumed that the woman's career can wait. Even if husbands are supportive, decisions made on a day-to-day basis often involve compromise on the woman's part. There often seems to be a pretext of why, for each minor event, it would be "easier" for the woman to compromise, especially when it involves children. Thus, in the end, many small compromises can lead to women losing their goals in the face of what appears to be an excellent support system. In my case, I found that standing my ground on each of the minor decisions felt petty and argumentative. It certainly would have been easier to give in each time. Ultimately, however, sticking to my position led to fewer arguments and a better relationship, as it established a fair balance. Indeed, I can now say that I have been fortunate in that successfully achieving this balance allowed me to have four children and that as they have been growing up, my husband has assumed an increasingly greater role in their day-to-day activities and the exigencies of their lives, which is not always the case for women in medicine. Further, if one were to ask him now, I am certain he would admit that my "forcing" him to share day-to-day childcare responsibilities has led to a type of fulfillment that he treasures.

For me, coping with the demands of my personal and professional life has been difficult in different ways at different stages of my career and at different ages. I suspect this is true for all women in medicine, particularly those who have achieved and function in leadership roles. When my children (who are now 18, 15, 12 and 9 years old) were younger, striking a workable balance was more stressful than it is now. That stress has been lessened because when we had our fourth child, my husband and I agreed that he would devote more time to the children. Because he is also a physician and our combined incomes allow us a very good standard of living, we have learned not to cut corners in solving the many needs of our children and our professional lives. We have adopted a philosophy of not being "pennywise and pound foolish." So, for example, if the babysitter we hired is sick and cannot take the children to school, we will call a taxi for them. We pay our babysitter more than the going rate in the market place rather than try to economize and face having to hire one babysitter after another. Another key factor that has allowed me to cope with the demands of balancing a professional and personal life is that I do not succumb to guilt — guilt that

I am not providing my children with enough time or love. I feel that my professional success and the salary that goes with it, the important work that I am able to do, along with my husband's contribution and the devotion and love that we have for our children, have provided our children with a standard of living, a home, role models and opportunities that far exceed those of the majority of people on this planet. Put in that perspective, I do not feel guilty over the time that I spend at work. My mother died when I was 12 years old and she was sick for most of my childhood, yet I still consider that my childhood was excellent, and my children's lives are that much better. I do manage to spend quite a bit of time with my family despite the pressures of work. I attend most of their productions at school, we take vacations together, and we talk and share ideas. Additionally, I believe that my children benefit from being proud of me when they hear from their friends, some of whose parents also work at M. D. Anderson, that I am an excellent physician. Over the years my children have had lots of positive feedback about me and have increasingly come to understand that the job I do is very worthwhile.

One example of this understanding occurred when my now-15-year-old son was 8 years old and was starring in a school production that I had told him I would attend. At the last minute I couldn't get out of the hospital in time to get there. A long-time patient of mine, with whom I had become very close, was in the hospital dying after 15 years in and out of remission from lymphoma. When we had first met, at the time of her diagnosis, her two sons were 8 and 9 years old and her primary goal was to live long enough to see them grow up. As she lay in the hospital, her boys were ages 22 and 23. Because I had been their mother's doctor and had bonded with the family and they with me, they wanted me to stay with their mother during her last hours. Later, when my young son expressed his disappointment about my absence at his school function, I explained the situation to him. In fact, he started crying and felt very strongly that I had made the best choice under the circumstances. I am quite sure that he identified with my patient's sons and their mother's situation, since he was the same age they had been when she first fell ill.

I personally feel very fortunate to have spent my career doing things that I really love and to have been successful at my efforts. I also feel fortunate that my success has been recognized, as reflected by the fact that I now lead one of the best, if not the best, early cancer clinical trials program in the nation and the world. Achieving this position can be attributed in part to my abilities and persistence, but other factors, including having good luck and the support of people around me and being in the right place at the right time, have played a part in forging success in my professional life. I am fortunate that all of those factors came together in a way that has allowed me to do what I set out to do so long ago. Most important, I am fortunate to have the privilege to do work that is meaningful and to have the opportunity to make an impact on a disease such as cancer.

I am often asked whether I have interests outside of work. I do, but to be frank, they are minor. My interests include skiing, running and reading. I have run the half-marathon thrice and will continue to do so yearly for as long as it is feasible. I tend to read books that relate to real life, such as biographies, rather than fiction, as I believe that real life is far more interesting. My major passion remains my family and children: Benjamin, who is 18 years old; Jonathan, 15; Rena, 12, and Tali, who was adopted at 14 months of age and is now 9. Although I never wanted children as a young woman, it turns out that despite my satisfaction and pride in my career and the good work that we do with cancer patients, my children top the list of what is truly important to me. I would have regretted not having them. The near-miss of almost forgoing this experience scares me when I think about how different and empty my life would have been without my children. I made a conscious decision to have children because Philip, the man I married and to whom I am still married, wanted children and it would not have been fair to him to marry him and not agree to have a family. I believe many women with demanding professional lives have conflicts about having children. There is such a strong bond between a mother and her children, but that bond is nearly impossible to understand *before* a woman has children. To have an active career *and* children requires a flexible and understanding husband. A firm partnership with and help from your husband is necessary. It is also best, I believe, not to be bullied by the many perceived needs of the children, particularly in today's child-centered culture. Their needs are, of course, important, but centering your entire life around them ultimately helps neither the children nor the parents.

My three older children are similar. They are all good kids and all extroverted, but serious *and* social, with both feet on the ground. In fact, they are quite similar to their dad. Benjamin, a first-year student at college, is serious and interested in law, economics and business. Jonathan loves the theater, but I truly believe despite his current disavowals that he will end up in medicine. He is very caring and wants to do something meaningful for his career. Rena may take that same path. She is almost obsessed with books about youngsters and young adults with serious illnesses. Tali is the most like me, especially as I was as a child. She is conservative, reserved, shy and introverted, with a great love of horses. She is also very artistic. It is fascinating to watch each child grow and develop into an individual and to help them to develop the best possible life. I believe it is necessary to communicate with your children about real issues, careers, children and feelings, and my husband and I have made this a priority in our lives.

In summary, I believe that I have been blessed in many ways. I have worked in a field that I enjoy, at a great institution doing a job that is meaningful. I have a wonderful, warm and loving family. Looking back, besides simple good luck, the main things that I may have contributed to build this good fortune were a clear vision of what I wanted out of life and an absolute dogged persistence to get there.

Guillermina Lozano, Ph.D.

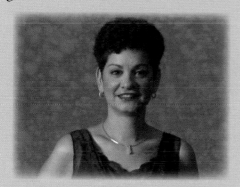

**Professor and Chair of Genetics
Mattie Allen Fair Research Chair**

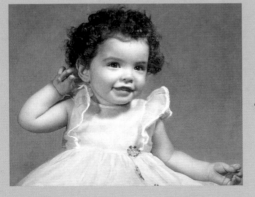

Gigi shows her winning smile at age 1.

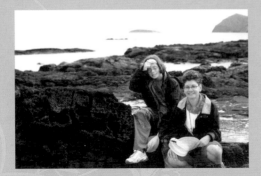

Daughter Rebecca enjoyed visiting the Galapagos Islands with Gigi in 2004.

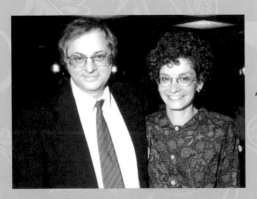

Gigi was happy to see her postdoctoral advisor Arnold Levine, Ph.D., when he attended a conference at M.D. Anderson in 1995.

As a child growing up in a Hispanic family, I never dreamed I would be an academician, much less a scientist. My father was born in Marin, Nuevo Leon, Mexico, and my mother, on a farm in El Porvenir. Neither of my parents had a high school education. They were married in Mexico and moved to East Chicago, where I was born a year later. My father worked in the steel mills, and my mother raised six children. Growing up, I was totally consumed with learning English (I spoke no English when I started school), learning the ways of a new culture, and in general trying to "fit in." Even then, I knew that I loved learning and loved a challenge.

In grade school, I found science to be the most boring subject I ever took. I thought we spent too much time regurgitating facts, and I hated science projects because I never had any ideas or the materials to put a project together. (In contrast, I thought math was fun, as it was very logical.) However, once I got to high school, my views about science changed completely. Originally, I was to attend the local high school, but, since racial riots were occurring there, my father instead sent my younger sister and me to an outstanding Catholic high school, Bishop Noll. As a sophomore there, I had an amazing biology teacher who opened up a world for me that I had not even known existed. I still remember learning how cells divide and how genes are inherited! The following year, we moved to a nice neighborhood, and again I was scheduled to attend the local high school. Excited about all that I was learning, I wanted to continue at Bishop Noll, but the tuition payments were hard on the family. So, I found a job preparing and cooking food at a local restaurant with the help of a friend and paid my own tuition and transportation so that I could remain at Bishop Noll. As a junior, I had another great teacher in chemistry — and I was hooked! I *knew* then that I wanted to do something in science.

The summer before my senior year of high school, we moved again, this time to McAllen, Texas. My father was losing his eyesight and hearing because of Usher's syndrome, an inherited autosomal recessive disease, and wanted to be close to his family in Mexico. The schools in south Texas were not as good as in Chicago, and I spent a depressing senior year rehashing a lot of what I had already learned. Even my physics class was easy.

I attended a local college in south Texas, Pan American University, thinking that I was going to be a biology teacher. I had no idea what careers were available for scientists — much less that anyone could actually do research. I was invited to join the honors program, and one of the requirements was to produce an honors thesis, so I began searching for a biology mentor to help me with my research. Although many of my teachers were not enthusiastic about mentoring a student, a new young faculty member, Terry Schultz, took me under his wing. The laboratory was small but brimming with activity. Dr. Schultz made me aware of other research opportunities, and so I applied and was accepted to the summer research program at the Oak Ridge National Laboratory in the summer of my junior year. That summer, I spent hours in the lab isolating frog embryos and examining the first steps of development. A few months later, I finished my honors thesis and graduated *magna cum laude*.

Even after graduation from college, I still had no reason at that point to think that I would ever be a successful scientist. As the oldest of six children — and a girl — born to immigrant parents from Mexico, I was expected to grow up, get married and have children. Furthermore, I had attended a school few had ever heard of and had not read my first scientific journal until I was a junior in college (and that was only because I went to the UT library in Austin when my parents and I went to pick up my brother, a freshman at UT). After graduation, I bucked my parents' wishes that I stay home in Texas. I remember having a long conversation with my father. I told him that just because he had decided to spend the rest of his life in south Texas didn't mean that I had to do the same. I think it was my thirst to learn, to do research and to see the world that motivated me to take this bold step. I had caught a glimpse of that exciting world, and there was no turning back.

I spent the summer after graduation at the National Institutes of Health in Bethesda, Maryland. I was thrilled! My supervisor, Gabriel Vogeli, chose my application from a table strewn with others because he liked my name. He picked me up at the bus stop in Bethesda, and I stayed with his family for a couple of days until I found a place to live. At the NIH, I interacted with many famous scientists and was always in the lab. Restriction enzymes had just become available, and I ordered my own! I learned molecular biology and was co-author on a manuscript (my first!). These opportunities cemented my love for research.

After that summer at the NIH, I began graduate school at the Oak Ridge National Laboratory. My academic background had not prepared me for the rigors of a graduate program, and I was always playing catch up. On the first day of graduate school, we learned that the graduate program had accepted too many students and could only afford to keep half of us. After that, learning became very competitive. (To this day, I prefer a nurturing environment instead of cut-throat competition.) After that first year of graduate school, I examined my options. I spent another summer at the NIH in the same laboratory and then accepted a job as a research technician at the Max Planck Institute for Biochemistry in Munich, Germany.

This was for me a time of exploring new professional and personal horizons. I got my first passport and then lost my plane ticket and had to call Dad to ask if I could use his credit card to buy another one. (Fortunately, he said that I could.) I spent two wonderful years in Germany discussing research projects with students, postdoctoral fellows and faculty (everyone wanted to practice their English); editing manuscripts; and learning new techniques. I gained valuable research experience. Importantly, I also pursued my passion for traveling. I traveled Europe with new friends and visited Paris for the first time, Berlin behind the Iron Curtain, and Czechoslovakia (as it was then known). I drank fabulous wines in Bordeaux and walked the streets of Venice and Rome. I hiked and climbed the Alps any chance I could get. Reaching the top of a peak after so much labor to get there is one of life's most rewarding experiences, not unlike a scientist's struggles and achievements in the lab. In between all these adventures, I worked hard and published my first paper as a first author. I had the best boss — Peter Mueller, still a close friend — and he encouraged me to return to school. He was confident that I had the intelligence, drive and skills to obtain a Ph.D. and succeed as a scientist. I was having the time of my life, so returning to graduate school was not an easy decision for me to make. Yet I realized that I really, really liked research and also that creative opportunities for technicians were limited. I had too many ideas of *my own*. I decided to apply to one school, Rutgers University, to work with one person, Bjorn Olsen, in the same area that I had published in, the extracellular matrix. I wanted to spend as little time as possible in graduate school, as I was eager to move forward to the next phase of my life. Three years and two months after starting graduate school, I defended my thesis.

I have many wonderful memories of graduate school. When I presented my findings from studies I had done in Germany at a group meeting, one of the professors thought that I was a new postdoc! I studied with friends and did well in my classes. I even passed my language exam in German. I met a wonderful older couple who became my New Jersey parents and fed me Sunday dinner on a regular basis. I also met my husband, Gregory May, a postdoctoral fellow at the time, in journal club. We were married less than a year after our first date.

Princeton was my next stop. I was surprised to get many offers for a postdoctoral fellowship but finally decided that it would be "cool" to manipulate the DNA of a mouse to understand the biology of oncogenes. So, I accepted a postdoctoral fellowship at Princeton University with Arnold Levine, who was doing research in that area. I had a long commute, but fortunately, my husband Greg was and is a great cook and had dinner ready most nights when I got home. At Princeton, I met many wonderful students, postdoctoral fellows and faculty.

My first few months as a postdoctoral fellow were difficult. I had completely changed fields and was on a steep learning curve. I was learning to manipulate fertilized one-cell mouse embryos and to implant them into pseudo-pregnant females. I soon realized that the two people I needed to learn from were not talking to each other. Then, a Southern blot of my mouse-tail DNA samples disappeared from my bench. I diplomatically plowed ahead.

By 1987, my husband had already spent four years as a postdoctoral fellow and was ready to move on, whereas I had spent less than two years as a postdoc. His best offer was in Houston. Again, I got offers for postdoctoral positions in Houston but knew that I would be looking for a permanent position as an independent scientist in the near future. Then I learned that the chief of the laboratory I had worked in at the NIH, Benoit de Crombrugghe, was moving to Houston as chair of the Department of Molecular Genetics at M. D. Anderson Cancer Center. I met with him and applied for a position. Dr. de Crombrugghe was very supportive and initially offered me a 'super' postdoctoral position but since I wanted to write a grant, I asked whether it could be a faculty position instead. I guess I must have impressed him since he offered me an instructor position and promised me promotion to assistant professor after one year. I grabbed the opportunity, and we (my husband and I *and* the mice) moved to Houston.

The hardest and most rewarding thing I have ever done is set up my own laboratory. Independent scientists are not trained to manage people, money and resources, yet that is exactly what we have to do to succeed. One of the first major decisions I made was to fire the first two people who worked for me. One was a technician assigned to me who had no molecular biology experience and had previously worked in a laboratory that allowed her to leave early. I was willing to train her, but she showed no interest in learning molecular biology. The second person, whom I had hired to work with the mice, had 10 years of experience with animals but could not tell the difference between a male and a female mouse. I realized that if my career depended on these two individuals, I would be "sunk." I tried to work with the technician to improve her performance, but it became obvious that she did not want to work with me, and she eventually transferred to another laboratory. I eventually fired the animal technician. Firing someone is never easy, but sometimes it is essential to move forward.

The next major challenge was writing my first grant. I read the NIH instructions 10 times (literally). Then, before submitting the grant, I had other scientists read my first draft and was crushed by their criticisms, although they were warranted. I worked hard to revise the application, and it paid off. The application was funded, and I was off and running.

My new technician, the daughter of an old family friend (the one who got me that first job in Chicago), was fresh out of college and eager to learn. I hired my first postdoctoral fellow from Canada, and a surgical oncology fellow and my first graduate student joined the lab. It was a great research team, and my ideas started moving forward. Our first major discovery was that the tumor suppressor p53 was a transcription factor. I still remember holding the film in the hallway and thinking, "Wow, I know something that no one else in the world knows!" Three years after setting up the laboratory, we published our first paper in *Science*.

Compared to setting up the laboratory, the rest of my career has been relatively easy. I was tenured and promoted to associate professor. The laboratory grew, and eventually we were all contributing ideas to the research effort. I enjoy being surrounded by smart people and love batting around ideas with my team. The most fun I have is the thrill of discovering something new. I continued to write grants and publish our findings. I was offered the chance to lead a section in Cancer Genetics at M. D. Anderson and jumped at the opportunity to bring in new faculty and create a cohesive program. I have a one-step-at-a-time philosophy. I start small, learn, build, and then steamroll down the hill. Last year, my section became the Department of Cancer Genetics with me at its helm. This year, we merged with the Department of Molecular Genetics and became the Department of Genetics. Now I have been at M. D. Anderson for more than 20 years. I have wonderful colleagues, and I have been given the opportunity to grow.

I sometimes think about why I have been so successful. My scientific curiosity tops the list of reasons. I have always wanted to learn new things; for example, when I read a manuscript, I have hundreds of questions. Also, my mentors (all men) gave me the confidence I needed to go to the next step. I never planned too far ahead because I had no idea what opportunities were available to me, but when an exciting opportunity arose, I was quick to take it. I have been very lucky and have always done my best. And while not all of my decisions have been right, I have always learned from their consequences.

My strong and supportive family is another major reason for my success. My husband, Greg, is also a scientist, and we often discuss ideas on the way home from work or at the dinner table. My daughter, Rebecca, was born while I was an assistant professor, and even though she is now a teenager, she still keeps me sane. If not for her and Greg, I would work non-stop and probably would have burned out by now. Fortunately, both Greg and Rebecca love to travel as much as I do, and we have traveled the world.

I think it is vitally important to have interests outside the laboratory. Besides enjoying my family, I grow orchids and play the piano. It is very rewarding to nurture a plant into full bloom, and it takes much less time than nurturing a graduate student. I learned to play the piano as an adult; it was something that I had always wanted to do as a child, but my family could not afford lessons, let alone a piano. I find playing the piano to be very refreshing because it frees my mind from all other issues. When I play, I must concentrate very hard on which hand or fingers to use, how hard to press the keys, and whether the notes are connected or staccato. While I am playing, I cannot think about anything else.

Another reason for my success is that I am somewhat competitive. O.K., I am *very* competitive and always have been. When one of my teachers in high school said that boys were smarter than girls, I set out to prove him wrong, and I did — I had the top grade in that class all year. Years later, when I learned that another researcher had already submitted a competing manuscript, a postdoctoral fellow and I wrote and submitted our manuscript in one weekend. Also, I have learned to focus on the important issues, and I try not to get stuck in the mire of every detail. This lesson is important not only in scientific inquiry but also in the administrative realm. Any one of those jobs can be overwhelming. Identifying the most important criteria for success is critical to achieving it. For example, I learned early on that funding and publishing were two essential aspects of my career. They trump everything else I do. I, therefore, spend the most productive hours of my day reading and writing.

I think that to be successful in any endeavor, it is very important to know your strengths and weaknesses and to play to your strengths. I am well organized, a skilled writer and a logical thinker, but I know my weaknesses and I am constantly learning to overcome them. For example, tooting my own horn is not something I do well. I have always thought that my accomplishments would speak for themselves and that everyone would recognize and acknowledge what I have done. However, I have learned that in this busy world I need to remind others of my accomplishments, although I still don't like to do it.

Juggling personal and professional demands is not easy. Fortunately, I have a husband who contributes substantially to the chores at home, including doing the grocery shopping and all the cooking. Most nights, we have dinner as a family and catch up on each other's day. I often take work home with me, and my daughter loves that we are both doing "homework." I try to limit my travel to once a month (though it doesn't always work out that way), and I have become choosey about the meetings I attend and the invitations I accept — I have learned to say no to many. And when I am all stressed out and overwhelmed, I take a deep breath, leave my watch at home, and decide which meetings I can afford to skip and which deadlines are soft ones. Finally, I don't take myself too seriously, and I laugh with friends as often as I can.

Karen H. Lu, M.D.

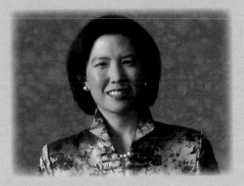

Professor of Gynecologic Oncology
H.E.B. Professorship in Cancer Research

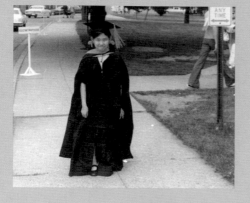

Karen tried on the cap and gown her mother wore to receive her master's degree.

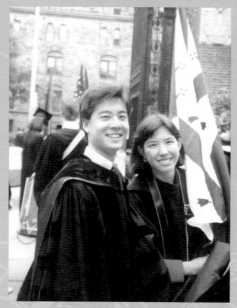

Both Karen and husband Charles Lu, M.D., received medical degrees from Yale University School of Medicine in 1991.

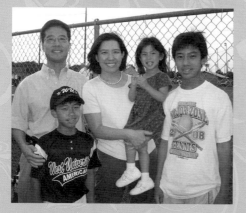

Ned, 10, at left, and David, 14 can count on parents Charles and Karen, holding Kate, 2, to cheer for their various sports teams.

ow I ended up where I am today is much clearer when examined in hindsight. Now, the choices I made that led me to my life's work as a gynecologic oncologist with a particular interest in hereditary cancers make sense. These choices were, in fact, not as random as they seemed at the time that each decision had to be made. Values that I hold and that were instilled in me — love of family, importance of the academic pursuit, joy of teaching — all guided those decisions.

I was born and raised in Baltimore, Maryland. My parents came from mainland China via Hong Kong to the United States to attend college and graduate school in the 1950s. Both came from scholarly families in China, and perhaps my commitment to academics comes from them. My paternal grandfather was a professor of chemistry who was educated at Johns Hopkins University. He was among a group of Chinese young men educated in the United States with scholarship funds established by the United States after the Boxer Rebellion. My maternal grandfather, a professor of economics, was educated in France. He later served as the head of China's legislature before the Communist regime, but I knew him only as the kind grandfather who played card games with me and gave me Juicy Fruit gum.

More recently, I have thought about the genetic link to my maternal grandmother. She was one of the first female graduates of Beijing University in the 1920s, where she majored in physics. Thereafter, she raised four children, served as a political wife, moved her family around China during the war in the early 1940s, and finally fled China for Hong Kong. I remember my mother telling me that while the rest of the family stayed in Hong Kong, my grandmother went to Malaysia by herself to teach college physics in order to support the family. Did she think about career goals? Did she worry about achieving the right balance of work and family life? Did she experience difficulties in academics because she was a woman? What I wouldn't give to be able to have a conversation with her now!

In contrast to my parents' and grandparents' dramatic lives, my childhood growing up in Baltimore was certainly less eventful. My immigrant parents believed that the route to success for their children in this new country was through education, so my brother and I went to traditional college prep schools in Baltimore (boys' school for him, girls' school for me). I loved attending an all-girls school because we were encouraged in every possible way. There was never any question that my classmates and I could achieve whatever we wanted to achieve, academically or otherwise. Contrary to the stereotype of Chinese parents, my parents never pushed me or my older brother academically, although I *do* think the ethic and value of scholarly pursuit was always present for us. We were both encouraged equally. The only time that my older brother felt any pressure from my dad was his gentle encouragement of my brother to go to Johns Hopkins, since both my dad and grandfather had been students there. Since my brother chose to go there for his undergraduate studies and for his Ph.D., by the time I was deciding about colleges, the familial obligation had been fulfilled, and I headed north to Harvard.

In college, I was a biochemistry major; I chose that major partly because it led me to a smaller community within the university that was fairly nurturing. We had one-on-one tutorials with faculty and were required to do a project with a mentor that would lead to a thesis. I worked with David Williams, an M.D.-Ph.D. doing a pediatric hematology-oncology fellowship at Children's Hospital. He was from the Midwest and was smart, hard working and kind. Ultimately, what I valued from my experience with him was that he was an incredibly decent human being with equal passions for the research he was doing, for the pediatric cancer patients he was caring for and for his young family. I learned about the dedication that research involves (lots of weekends and nights with mice), and I learned about the value of scientific pursuit in medicine. Looking back now, it seems that experience must have influenced my decision to combine my own passions: for caring for women with gynecologic cancers, for translational research, and for my husband and three children.

One of my best experiences in college was meeting my future husband, Charlie. We grew up together in college and were great friends. We dated all through college, went our own ways for a few years, and then started dating again when we both were at Yale Medical School. When it was time to make decisions about matching for residencies, it seemed for us an easy decision to get married and enter into the "couples match." A "couples match" allows two people to merge their prospects together in the lottery that determines where medical students will do their residencies. It is a good test in negotiation and compromise for couples, and we had a relatively easy time deciding on our choices. By the time we got married at the end of medical school, Charlie and I had known each other for almost 10 years. I tell my sons that they need to really, *really* know someone before they get married, and I use our 10-year standard for their reference. I may have to revise my advice, but my point is this: having a long history with someone makes facing the challenges of life easier.

We ended up in Boston for residency — Charlie in Internal Medicine and me in Obstetrics and Gynecology. I loved residency. After all that coursework, this was the time when you really learned to be a doctor, and I loved all of it: delivering babies, surgery, clinic. My colleagues were fun, and the ones who weren't provided fodder for good humor. We worked like dogs, but it was easy to feel a sense of instant gratification. I do remember tough times of getting no sleep at night and then having to face a busy clinic the next day. My motto for nights on call was: you had to sleep or you had to eat. If you couldn't do one, you had to do the other.

During the end of my second year of residency, I had to start thinking about whether to apply for a fellowship in one of the four subspecialties in obstetrics/gynecology. I definitely had a preference for subspecializing, as I didn't think that being a general obstetrics/gynecology physician, which usually meant private practice, fit me well. But what specialty? Urogynecology had interesting vaginal surgery, but I had a hard time getting passionate about urinary incontinence. The reproductive endocrinology and infertility attendings did interesting laparoscopic surgery, but I wasn't particularly passionate about infertility or endocrinology. That left gynecologic oncology. Not for the faint of heart, this field is unique in that it combines expertise in complex surgeries with expertise in chemotherapy. For a resident, this is one of the most exhausting yet most exhilarating and gratifying rotations. At the time, it was not the obvious choice for me, but, looking back, I cannot imagine a more suitable field. I am *passionate* about working with women who have gynecologic cancers.

The fellowship was three years, and, since my husband had started his medical oncology fellowship in Boston a year earlier, it made sense for me to remain in Boston for my fellowship, too. And as much as I enjoyed my residency, I enjoyed my fellowship more. The first year was a lab year, and I worked in Sam Mok's lab. Those in the field of ovarian cancer research know him for his accomplishments in understanding the molecular pathogenesis of disease. I had not thought seriously about lab work since college, but Sam brought out the latent molecular biologist in me. During that year, I understood the power of clinicians working with basic scientists. Sam had expertise, techniques and tissues to study ovarian cancer. Sam gave all new fellows in the lab a project that was already under way. After completing this initial project, we could start thinking about our own ideas for studies. This is what I loved. I could think of endless clinical scenarios in which having a molecular biology answer would really be helpful. Sam taught me the importance of having a tissue and serum bank. Because those resources were in place, I was able to ask and answer clinical questions using molecular biology and do it within a short period of time. Writing and submitting abstracts, assembling posters (back then, there was a lot more cutting and pasting), putting together PowerPoint presentations, and learning to write, re-write, and (again) re-write a manuscript are skills that I learned during my fellowship. You only have to do these things once or twice before the tasks become easier and less daunting. I can unequivocally state that my style of mentoring clinical gynecologic oncology fellows today derives directly from the way in which I learned from Sam and others during my fellowship.

It was also during my fellowship that I developed my interest in hereditary cancer syndromes. BRCA1 and BRCA2 had recently been cloned, and there were plenty of clinical questions that needed answering. I remember during my clinical year taking care of a woman who was petrified that she would get ovarian cancer. Multiple women in her family had died of this disease, and she had recently found out that she carried a mutation in BRCA1. Although she was only in her mid-30s, we were going to remove her ovaries, and she was happy about it. Her surgery, done laparoscopically, was uneventful, and she went home the same day. A week later, we heard from the pathologist that both her ovaries and fallopian tubes showed microscopic pre-cancerous changes. But, unlike her female relatives, whose ovarian cancer had been diagnosed at stage 3 or 4 (when it is already widely disseminated, which is typically when it is diagnosed), she had her ovaries removed just as the cancerous process was beginning and, thus, was able to escape the fate of her female relatives. This experience made the power of the discovery of the BRCA1 and BRCA2 genes very real and vivid to me.

After spending 16 years in New England for college, medical school and training, I was hoping that we would move home to Baltimore for our first real jobs. Johns Hopkins and the National Cancer Institute (NCI) were obvious choices, so very early on (the end of my second year in fellowship), we approached our respective oncology departments there to ask about opportunities. However, it was entirely obvious, from a few phone calls and one interview, that neither was going to be a good fit for us.

Soon afterward, right before the start of my third year of fellowship, Charlie attended a meeting in Colorado and ran into a friend who had recently started work as an attending at M. D. Anderson Cancer Center in Houston. Was Charlie starting to look for a job? Would he like to have dinner with Dr. Waun Ki Hong the next evening? I remember the phone conversation with my husband after he had met with Dr. Hong — great job, great opportunity, great institution. Charlie flew down to Houston very soon afterward for an interview, and I began to pay attention when he came home and asked me if we could fax my resume to M. D. Anderson to see if there was a job opening in gynecologic oncology. From there, things progressed fairly quickly.

When Charlie went for his second interview, I went along. Although there was no formal job opening for me, at that time the department and program were expanding their translational research program in ovarian cancer. I had already secured funding from the American Gynecologic and Obstetric Society to do three years of translational research training. The enthusiasm of Charlie's three friends from Harvard was consistent and overwhelming: for junior faculty wanting academic opportunities, M. D. Anderson was *the* place to be. My lesson from this experience was this — start early to look for jobs in places that you really think you want to go. If it doesn't work, keep an open mind. It is likely that the best opportunity may surprise you.

I remember one of my mentors in the fellowship program saying that you need to leave the institution where you trained so that you can grow up. If you stay, your attendings will see you as their trainee, and, worse, you will always feel like a trainee. I don't know whether that is always the case, but I *do* think it is good advice. It was healthy for me to leave Boston and my comfort zone. I learned that I could meet a new set of colleagues, find collaborators and mentors, figure out the way to a new operating room, and establish myself.

Two very fortunate events that occurred early in my career have defined the direction of my research and clinical interests. First, I came from my fellowship with an interest in hereditary cancers. A significant portion of my research as a fellow was devoted to ovarian cancer and BRCA1 and BRCA2. When I came to M. D. Anderson, I wanted to continue that interest but found out that there were fewer than 10 families with known mutations — not enough raw material to do any substantive research. I remember a chance encounter with Dr. Patrick Lynch, who led the registry for Hereditary Non-polyposis Colorectal Cancer (HNPCC), now referred to as Lynch syndrome. He said, "You know, we can never get any gynecologists to study Lynch syndrome." What lay in front of me was a rich registry and expertise in a hereditary cancer syndrome in which women had an equal and significant risk of developing endometrial and colon cancer as well as a smaller but significant risk of ovarian cancer. I consider myself fortunate to have fallen into such an opportunity.

The second fortuitous event occurred when my colleague Dr. Russell Broaddus and I found out about a Request for Applications (RFA) from the NCI to conduct an endometrial cancer chemoprevention study in women with HNPCC. There had been very little studied on endometrial cancer and Lynch syndrome in general, but the goal was to examine two agents known to be effective in preventing endometrial cancer in the general population: oral contraceptives and progesterone. To really get a study like this done, two components would be necessary: 1) a registry of Lynch syndrome families from which to draw eligible women, and 2) knowledge of molecular biomarkers relevant to endometrial cancer that could be used as surrogate endpoints. I think we believed that this was something we *had* to do — where else was there such an established Lynch syndrome registry and investigators interested in endometrial cancer prevention? In addition, Russell knew a group at the UT Medical School that was studying the molecular effects of estrogen on post-menopausal endometrium in the context of hormone replacement therapy. Wouldn't it make sense to look at some of these same genes in endometrial cancer, which is believed to result from too much estrogen in the endometrium? There was a fantastic opportunity to examine some of these novel genes as biomarkers. All the necessary pieces were in place to apply for this grant, but there was one catch. Neither of us had applied for this type of grant before, and the deadline was only four weeks away. I call this our "soup to nuts" grant submission. Russell and I had no expertise in putting together a budget or in assembling a consortium of other institutions, which required even more paperwork and more complicated budgeting. What we *did* have was youthful enthusiasm and help from Dr. Lynch's team, which had recently completed a colon cancer chemoprevention study. We ended up getting the grant and gaining a lot of confidence along the way. This year, five years later, we completed accrual to this study. It took sheer force of will and a number of very dedicated individuals to complete this trial, and ours is one of the few, if not the only, gynecologic chemoprevention study for a hereditary cancer syndrome that has actually completed accrual.

The same youthful enthusiasm that went into this first grant re-surfaced when we began to consider submitting a uterine SPORE grant. I remember Russell, Mai Dinh (our project coordinator) and I meeting with one of our most respected mentors, Dr. George Stancel, who is dean of our UT Graduate School for Biomedical Sciences. We had lunch with him and proudly pronounced that we wanted to put a uterine SPORE grant together. He gave us really sound advice: don't do it. I give full credit to Russell and Dr. Tom Burke for saying, "Let's just try it anyway." The deadline for submission only gave us eight weeks to focus on preparing the grant, but, frankly, after that chemoprevention grant went in, nothing seemed impossible. Because of Congressional budget delays, we didn't find out until some 18 months after submission that the grant would be funded. By then, we just wanted the money and to get started with the research. My continued love for the research process has grown with the growth of the uterine cancer program, both at our institution and nationwide. Our success has been partly due to bringing in expertise from very different disciplines to focus on a cancer that has been really understudied. The other key to our success has been to encourage and draw in enthusiastic young scientists.

Looking back, I am surprised that I never considered the work-life balance more carefully as I made my career decisions. I chose what most would consider a time-intensive specialty because I liked it. Having children was a given, and we planned as best we could. In my third year of residency, I had a non-clinical six-week rotation, which I used for my first maternity leave. Our second child was supposed to come during my non-clinical year of fellowship, but perfect planning doesn't always happen. Because I was a busy clinical fellow and because I wanted to honor a promise to my senior fellow that he could attend an important conference, I went back to work two weeks after my second son was born. I approached each of my maternity leaves by taking extra call while pregnant, trading favors, and fulfilling my job when I returned from leave. It is a delicate balance to have children during medical training or even as an attending. I respected my colleagues and didn't want to ever feel that I wasn't pulling my weight.

As for that last child, I had been on staff for six years, had been promoted to associate professor, and at 41 was considered by the standards of my field to be of "advanced maternal age." We had finally cleared our house of all the baby paraphernalia, since our boys were 12 and 8. I tell people that we needed a shot of excitement into our well-balanced life. Our daughter has provided that, and, after so many years without an infant, she reminded me how difficult it is for working women to have babies. For us, what has always worked was having lots of help, including a live-in nanny and my parents, who take turns coming to Houston. Since my father is retired, he spends weeks at a time with us here. He drives the morning carpool for the boys and in the afternoon takes them to tennis, baseball or piano lessons. At their games and tournaments, he is their biggest fan. My mother still teaches, and she comes to visit and help out when she can. I know I could not be where I am today without their help. Besides my husband and parents, there are other key individuals who help make it possible for me to do the work that I do. All working women need to understand the value of their assistants; I know I would be nowhere without mine, Jeannette Upshaw.

I grew up with parents and teachers who assumed I would choose a life's work and pursue it passionately. Balancing the commitments of work *and* family is difficult. Thus, choosing what you do in life becomes that much more important. I believe that if you have a true passion for the things you choose to pursue, whether personal or professional, the rewards will be well worth the effort. So far, it's been that way for me.

Funda Meric-Bernstam, M.D.

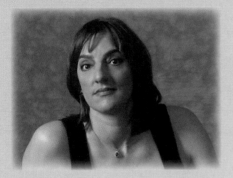

Associate Professor of Surgical Oncology

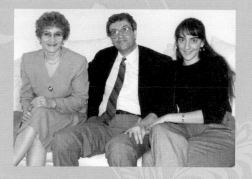

Funda and her parents, Gulser (left) and Ilhan Meric (center), on Thanksgiving Day, in Bethesda, Maryland, 1994.

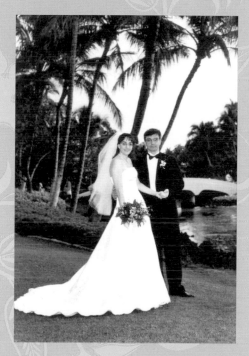

Funda and Elmer Bernstam were married in 2003 on the Big Island, Hawaii.

(Photo courtesy of Joyce Haverkate, Zac's Photo)

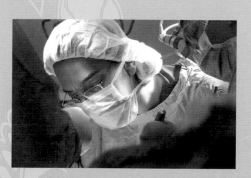

As a physician-scientist, Funda combines conducting translational research with providing surgical expertise to breast cancer patients.

(Photo by Karen Hensley)

I am the only child of two professors of finance, which ensured that I would never overvalue money or pursue a career in business. However, my choice of an academic career appears to have been genetically predetermined. Even when our family went on vacation, my parents were planning their next paper together. Also, it was quite clear (to me) that academic success led to trips to exotic locations. I am still not sure whether my parents travel for work or work for travel. In any case, they travel constantly, and, therefore, it appears that they are successful.

Apparently, I declared my interest in medicine at age four when I fell off of a radiator and split my lower lip. After the doctor had sutured my lip, I announced to my grandmother that I, too, wanted to be a doctor. That remained my goal throughout childhood and led me to make some strange requests (such as for an anatomy model for my 13th birthday). I briefly considered other career options. In junior high, I considered a career with Charlie's Angels or Jacques Cousteau. In high school, I very seriously considered physics and electrical engineering. I finally settled on academic surgical oncology, a career to which I appear to be well suited. Still, since I am generally a happy person, I probably also would have been happy as a Charlie's Angel or in many other careers.

My parents have always been pathologically supportive of me. I suppose many parents think that their children are the best, the smartest and the most successful. But my parents constantly remind me (and anyone else who will listen) of their conviction. My father tells his students, gas station attendants and random grocery store employees about his amazing daughter. Although English is my parents' second language, they are able to maintain a constant stream of superlatives. In fact, not a single day goes by without my mother telling me how much prouder she is of me today than yesterday or the day before. Perhaps this is one of the reasons I still talk to her every day. This positive reinforcement has served me well — but more about that later.

I moved around a lot as a child, which I think made me tougher, more flexible and adaptable to change. My parents came to the United States from Turkey to pursue their Ph.D.s in finance. I was born in the United States but lived with my grandparents in Turkey while my mom was finishing her Ph.D. When I was 4 years old and had just learned Turkish, my mom finished her Ph.D., and I was moved back to the United States. By the time I was 8 years old, I had forgotten Turkish but had learned fluent English. Unfortunately, my parents' scholarship required them, and by extension, me, to return to Turkey. Then, when I was a junior in high school, we again returned to the United States for my parents' sabbatical. Shortly thereafter, I moved back to Turkey, where I finished high school and started medical school at Hacettepe University in Ankara. At the time, my parents were junior faculty in the United States. Four years later, my dad got tenure, so I returned to the United States to join my parents.

In Turkey, I attended three schools. I started second grade in a public school, but everything was in Turkish, so I can't really tell you much about those six months, since that was during one of my English-speaking periods. Then I went to a private school where math, science and English were taught in English. I learned much more at this school, and indeed, I did not have to work very hard to be one of the top students. Throughout junior high, my parents kept telling me that the smartest kids went to "Science High School." (Think "Fame," but for bookworms rather than aspiring performers.) Admission was based on results of an entrance exam; the 96 students with the top scores were sent to this government-run boarding school, which was on the top of a mountain near Ankara. There, I went from being the smartest kid in most classes to one among many smart kids. It quickly became apparent that I had to work hard to excel in this group. On the other hand, I was now the most athletic; it helped that I was a foot taller than any of the boys. Alas, my basketball career was discouraged by a rigorous academic schedule and a lack of heat in the gymnasium. I also became involved in theater and played the lead ("Jo") in a school production of "Little Women." I like to think that my brief time as a thespian made me more comfortable in front of an audience.

The pinnacle of my academic career came early. In Turkey, all graduating high school students who wish to attend university must take an entrance examination, somewhat similar to taking the SAT in the United States. In 1983, approximately 500,000 students in Turkey took the exam, and I had the top score. The press interviewed my parents and me, and this gave my father plenty of opportunity to discuss his favorite subject — me. In addition to providing my proverbial 15 minutes of fame, this external validation of my parents' praise gave me lasting confidence. To this day, my husband jokingly introduces me as "the smartest person in Turkey."

After completing the first four years of a premed-medical program in Turkey, I decided to join my parents in the United States. Yale Medical School will always have a special place in my heart because they took a chance on me — a student from a foreign school. The years I spent at Yale were some of the happiest and most fruitful of my life thus far. Yale has a unique educational system: Because all Yale students are above average, there is no need for grades, so we studied for ourselves rather than "to make the grade." I believe that this approach provided me with the foundation for lifelong learning.

In addition, Yale required every graduating student to write a thesis. That thesis was my first clinical research experience, produced my first publication, and got me addicted to academic medicine. I think that this along with other research experiences during medical school led me to pursue research in molecular biology. Consider this my plug for involving students in research — it's *not* a waste of time.

Residency in general surgery was a, shall we say, "unique" experience. I am sorry to report that the events of my residency are not accurately represented on "Grey's Anatomy." In my experience, there was more work, less romance and less camaraderie. Before the 80-hour workweek rules came into effect, a surgery residency could be summarized as five years spent in the hospital. Perhaps I exaggerate — there were some nights spent in my own bed. On a positive note, it was great surgical training that taught me to "operate in my sleep." In fact, every few years, the local paper would (again) "discover" that surgery residents were working more than 100 hours per week and do an "expose."

During residency, there were never enough hours in the day to get everything done. We were forced to learn how to be as efficient as possible and to prioritize and multitask, skills that I now use every day. My fear of missing something and getting yelled at by a chief resident was eventually replaced by the fear of missing something that could hurt a patient. To this day, I maintain an intense — maybe too intense — sense of personal responsibility for my patients. I often wake up in the middle of the night to double-check test results.

At one point, during one of my general surgery interviews I was told that if I were accepted into the residency program, my ovaries would "shrink to the size of raisins." This comment heightened my awareness of the degree of gender bias that existed in the field of surgery. Finally, I chose a residency program at the University of Michigan, which was considered at that time to be one of the "woman-friendly" programs. Alas, many of the female surgery residents who were ahead of me there are now pursuing other careers. On one occasion, when I was playing with a young patient, an attending physician commented, "If you weren't wasting time doing this doctor stuff, you could have a few of your own one day." Chief residents also were fond of mentioning that there was "too much estrogen on the team." To this day, I believe that an important difference between me and those women who did not finish the program was the endless supply of positive reinforcement that I received from my parents.

Then, after years of being encouraged to be "one of the boys," when the time came to apply for fellowships, I was advised by an attending surgeon to wear a skirt and get a feminine haircut for the interviews (as if these superficial efforts were needed on top of all my hard work, studies and accomplishments). However, I took the advice. I got into M. D. Anderson Cancer Center, the premier surgical oncology fellowship.

As residents, we were encouraged to do research. For those of us interested in academic careers, this meant a two-year hiatus from clinical training between the third and fourth years of the general surgery residency program. I chose to spend this time at the National Institutes of Health (NIH) in Bethesda, Maryland. I chose the NIH because of its reputation but also because I was sick of the cold winters in Michigan.

I joined a large laboratory where I was the only M.D. among 20 Ph.D.s. This was a completely new world with its own traditions, language and expectations. During the first few months, I only understood about 20 percent of what was said at lab meetings. To make matters worse, my boss suggested that I pursue a general area of study (the process of generating protein from RNA) and gave me little guidance. I was mostly left to my own devices. I had to choose, design and carry out my own research project. That was challenging because many of my colleagues in the lab did not believe that surgeons could (or should, for that matter) be successful scientists. Therefore, to many of them, helping me was an unwelcome distraction unlikely to lead to anything productive. Fortunately, this turned out to be a growth opportunity in disguise. At the end of my two years at NIH, I left with the confidence that I could ask and answer the critical questions in any field.

It may not be entirely surprising that I met my husband in a medical library. We started out rollerblading and jogging together. Next came the dancing, which turned out to be false advertising: By the time we started officially dating, he claimed to have developed two left feet. There was also another, more serious problem: I had already matched at M. D. Anderson, and he was planning to train in biomedical informatics at Stanford. I don't recommend long-distance relationships, but, after three years, if you are still together, you know it is meant to be. I am not just saying this because my husband is helping me write this chapter — he *truly* makes my life worth living. We are very different in some ways, and, yet, he completes me (as well as my sentences and paragraphs). In fact, we have written numerous grants and papers together.

Marriage changed my life. It helps me maintain perspective at work and decreases my propensity to bring work home. It caused me to learn how to cook and to ski and to forget how to ballroom dance … but I digress. Marriage gets me out of the hospital and onto a tennis court or jogging track and makes travels to exotic places more fun. I now see that it is important to maintain balance, and I believe that having a life outside of work increases productivity in the long run.

It was my honor and privilege to train at M. D. Anderson Cancer Center with some of the best surgical oncologists in the world. I guess that, as a faculty member here, I'm pretty much required to say that, but I *really do feel that way*, and I consider myself lucky to have joined this faculty.

I chose to focus my research and surgical practice on breast cancer because to me, it is the most interesting disease in the world. There are not enough pages in this book to fully describe all of the facets of breast cancer that I find fascinating. Let's just say that even with all we now know about this disease, thousands of women still die of it every year. It is hard to imagine another disease that is more compelling to a female scientist. Also, since many patients with breast cancer prefer a female surgeon, being a woman in this specialty is an asset rather than a liability.

I joined the M. D. Anderson faculty as a surgeon-scientist. That means that I spend half of my time treating breast cancer patients and half of my time doing research. Realistically, this means that I have two full-time jobs. Clinical work, especially surgery, rarely fits into allotted time slots. Similarly, there is always more to be done in the lab, always another question to be asked.

It takes a lot of hard work to succeed. While at Yale, I met the owner of a successful local hamburger stand. I thought he was lucky because he did not have to work as hard as we medical students did, but it turned out that his day began at 5 a.m. and didn't end until he closed the store at midnight, seven days a week. It seems that in all careers, the top people work very hard. My mom says, "If you want to be more successful than your neighbor, work six days a week. If you want to be more successful than everyone else, work seven days a week."

When I joined the M. D. Anderson faculty, I felt that I was well prepared to be a breast surgeon. However, I quickly discovered that none of my training really prepared me to manage a clinical or research team. It took me several years to create the productive research environment that I have today. I think that this is often the case; you're trained to do something, and, if you do it well, you're told to stop and do something else.

I had to come to understand that it is not my job to make everyone happy. Rather, I must create a productive, harmonious work environment in which happiness is possible. I also realized that it makes no sense to expect everyone to be like me. To be effective as a leader, I had to understand people better and had to leverage shared goals to inspire and motivate them.

In research, as in life, it's easy to get distracted by minutiae. If you want to succeed, you have to set ambitious goals and then work to achieve them. Don't sweat the small stuff; value quality over quantity. Your time and resources are limited, so focus on the truly important. This is an exciting time in biomedicine. We now have the technologies to address the big questions: How can we target the molecular causes of cancer? Can we personalize treatment to a given individual?

It is important to realize, however, that no single person can provide answers to such questions — these answers require collaborative efforts. Certainly, it is important to have one's own niche, whether in clinical work or in research, but it is more important to work well within a team. We must put our egos aside and collaborate for the greater good. Teamwork and coordinated research efforts allow us to do larger projects that have a greater and more immediate impact on patients' lives.

Finally, I believe that success is a journey, not a destination. My advice: Enjoy the trip.

Vivian H. Porche, M.D.

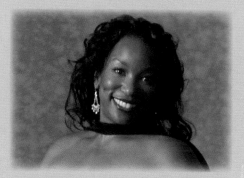

**Professor of Anesthesiology
and Pain Medicine**

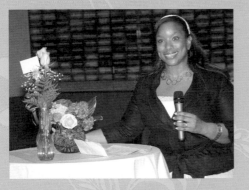

Vivian spoke at a 2007 reception honoring her for becoming the first African-American woman promoted to professor of anesthesiology and pain medicine at M.D. Anderson.

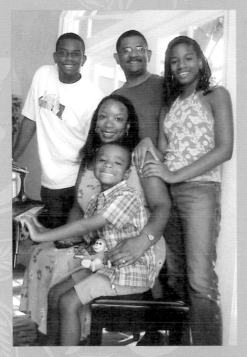

In a 2004 family photo, Vivian holds son Troy while husband Henry Porche stands between son Henry III and daughter Bobbi.

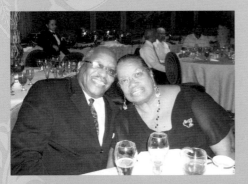

Vivian's parents, LaFrance and Bobby Harris, posed at a family member's wedding in 2007.

always dreamed of being a doctor, wife and mother but never imagined how difficult it would be to play these roles simultaneously. I had imagined myself living a June Cleaver-esque life, with spotless, well-behaved children who waited patiently at the breakfast table while I leisurely prepared the food. My ideal husband would also be at the table, reading the paper and giving sage advice to our inquisitive, charming children. After work, I would come home and happily greet the children before preparing dinner. After dinner, my husband and I would help the kids — who, of course, would be eager to learn and very smart — with their homework. At bedtime, the kids would snuggle into their beds, eagerly awaiting a story and a song that I would sing, sounding like Julie Andrews. After the kids fell asleep, I would have a stimulating conversation with my husband about world events before retiring for the night.

That scenario is truly a beautiful dream, but my *reality* is much different. On a typical morning, I am already on my way to work when the kids wake up. The kids get up, get dressed and eat a breakfast prepared by the nanny, who takes them to school. The nanny then cleans, shops, starts dinner and picks up the kids from school. By the time I come home 10 to 12 hours later, everyone is tired and irritable, and those charming children are nowhere to be found. Instead, I have three little people who do not want to do their homework and do not want to go to bed but do want to watch television. By the time they are in bed, it is too late for a story, and I am too exhausted to sing. My husband has arrived during this time, also wanting attention but not receiving any. Our conversation is short and mundane before we fall into bed. The weekends I am on call are not much better — actually, they are somewhat worse, since my nanny does not work weekends.

But before you feel too sorry for me, let me state that I love my life! I might not be living the dream from my childhood, but I *am* living a dream. I am married to my high school sweetheart, have three wonderful, brilliant children, and have a successful career. How did I get here, you ask? Well, in Langston Hughes' words, "Life for me ain't been no crystal stair." I have tripped, stumbled and fallen down while still "a-climbin' on, and reachin' landin's, and turnin' corners." Seeing the success of my mother and grandmother, even as they juggled their careers and family, has kept me on track. Equally important has been my faith and my determination; I knew then, as I know now, that I can do all things with God's help.

I am blessed to have two parents, LaFrance C. and Bobby W. Harris, and a set of grandparents, Joseph O. and Senora L. Williams, who earned college and postgraduate degrees. Growing up as an African-American female in a family where almost everyone had a professional degree helped me tremendously, even though I knew that this situation was not the norm. In my world, everyone went to college and women worked outside the home. Men also worked outside the home, but that was expected. What was "unexpected" was *how many jobs my own father held as we grew up.* Recognizing that he had to transition from giving orders to taking orders in his second and third jobs so that he could support his family made him almost *superhuman* in my eyes. Unyielding determination and perseverance are two of the many qualities my father demonstrated time and time again that have helped shape and mold me. Perhaps his productivity is a result of his own rearing by a mother who also assiduously worked at keeping her family together. Thus, when I was in junior high, at the beginning of desegregation, I was surprised to learn that many of my classmates had stay-at-home mothers. In my adolescent mind, I assumed that these women must have had some debilitating disease that prevented them from working. But with my mother and my friends' mothers as role models, I grew up seeing women work outside of the home and have successful careers.

My parents were both elementary school principals. My younger brother and I each attended a school in which one of our parents worked. That meant that everyone in school — teachers and students — knew us. Our every move was monitored. When we got into trouble, we were reprimanded at school *and* at home. While we were growing up, education was highly valued, and my parents fostered a love of discovery and learning in my brother and me. They also showed me how a strong faith can help one overcome any obstacle. I know this is true because God has taken care of my family and me through many storms, trials and troubles.

I always knew that I wanted to be a doctor, as I enjoy being an agent of change and helping others to be their best. I thought I wanted to be a cardiovascular surgeon until high school, when I had the opportunity to observe an open-heart surgery being performed. While watching, I saw that the anesthesiologist was an expectant mother and thought, "Hey, here's somebody who really is doing it all — being a doctor, a wife and a mother." (Of course, when I was in high school, I thought that anyone who was pregnant had to be married.) I began to realize that there were more possibilities, other than being a surgeon, than I had imagined!

College was fun. I studied, pledged Alpha Kappa Alpha sorority, dated and studied some more. I enjoyed most of my classes, volunteered at a hospital and was chairman of the African-American Culture Committee, and I did well in all of these activities. I also endured a class in which the professor actually taught that African-Americans are genetically inferior to whites. I may have had to listen to all of this, but I refused to receive any of what he said. I chose not to argue with him because I knew that I would not win. He would only lower my grade, which would give me a lower grade-point average that could possibly prevent me from entering medical school. This was a very deliberate decision — I knew what I wanted to do, and I decided to keep my eye on the prize.

Deciding on which medical school to attend was an easy choice for me. I wanted to stay close to home, and, fortunately, I had many schools to choose from. I applied to most of the schools in Texas, and, thankfully, was accepted to them all. I chose The University of Texas Medical School at Houston not only because of its proximity but also because of the wonderful opportunity for learning and discovery within the Texas Medical Center hospitals. I then began to consider how to achieve my additional goals of wife and mother and about how I could make my goals a reality. I methodically plotted out what I needed do first, then second, and so on, to achieve these goals. While planning, I realized two important things: First, I needed to have a boyfriend while in medical school, since I probably wouldn't have time to date, and, second, I would have to have children during my residency so I could be more marketable as an attending physician. Thank you, God, for that insight! I dated the man who would become my husband during my last semester of college and through most of medical school. We were married in my last year of medical school.

When I was interviewing at different anesthesiology residency programs, I had an encounter with the chair of anesthesiology at a program primarily made up of white men. When I asked him why there were no African-Americans on staff or in the program, he answered, "There aren't any qualified." I proceeded to tell him, much to his chagrin, that I was qualified, and I began to recite my accomplishments. Needless to say, I did not match there. However, that conversation has continued to stimulate me to always "aim for the stars to land above the trees." I matched with Baylor College of Medicine, my first choice for residency, and I was thrilled! Three years later, I had my first child during my residency. I decided to take three months of maternity leave before returning to work because I knew that those precious moments with my new baby could never be reclaimed.

Upon returning to work, I was thrust into the exciting world of cardiovascular surgery. As an anesthesiology resident, it was my duty to put the patients to sleep, keep them alive during the surgery, and wake them up at the end. I was still nursing my son when I returned to work, and I knew that I would need to use a breast pump during the day. I anticipated that my attending physician would be very understanding and allow me a little time during my breaks to pump before returning to the operating room. I was allowed to pump, but only when it was convenient for my attending, not when my breasts were full. This was not a problem until I had to stay in the operating room for a prolonged period because of a patient's critical condition. When the patient's condition improved, I was able to be relieved to pump, but only after watching my burgundy-colored scrubs turn pink because of all the milk that seeped through my shirt and after tolerating verbal abuse, which included several expletives, from my attending. Before I left the room, I asked my attending if he had any more suggestions to help me become better at my work. Well, that made him even angrier, and I was promptly dismissed to go on break. (During my career, this was one of many instances of enduring verbal abuse that included the use of the "n" word.) But I knew that whatever he or anyone else said to me was not going to deter me; I knew I was put in that place by a higher power. The lesson I learned that day was to keep a cool head when there is chaos all around. This skill has served me well through the years.

Dr. Melba Swafford, who was an attending physician during my cardiovascular rotation, was helpful then and continues to mentor and support me now. She was the only African-American anesthesiologist I saw during my residency and both of my fellowships. She was also the first African-American in her department. Melba may not be the head of a department or someone very famous, but her knowledge, dedication, expertise and compassion combined with her calm demeanor have shown me how to handle difficult situations. She taught me how to assert myself with quiet authority and dignity and made sure that I dotted my I's and crossed my T's! She encouraged me then and encourages me now to always be better than the rest and to never let them see you sweat.

I interviewed for my first job at M. D. Anderson Cancer Center while I was very pregnant with my second child. It was obvious when I met with my potential chairman that he was hesitant to hire his first female anesthesiologist — and one with two small children, at that. I fervently sold myself by reiterating that I was settled in my marriage and settled in my family, that I would not have any more children, that there was no need to worry about my going on maternity leave, and that besides we already had a nanny who would help with the kids. I left that meeting with a signed contract! Lesson learned from this: Have a plan and a back-up plan of action.

My first office mate arrived a few months after I started working. She had only been in practice a few years before coming to the institution. We became very friendly, especially since we both came from similar backgrounds: her parents, too, were educators; she had married her high school sweetheart, just as I had done; and she had two small children of her own. One day, she and I began to talk about our hopes and dreams, our families, and the moral influences of our upbringing. Then, a light bulb went off for my Caucasian friend. I will never forget how sincerely, and with a newfound realization, she said to me, "You people are just like us!" She then told me that her views of African-Americans had been shaped by negative images on television and that she had not personally known anyone like me. From then on and to this day, we have built a lasting friendship based on mutual respect, admiration and similarities.

One other colleague, an older white man, also changed his opinion of me after working and interacting with me. Before I even entered the operating room, I had been told that one of the men on staff was not happy that I was hired. "They hired another woman," he complained, "and this one has little kids. She will never be at work." Well, I heard that and I knew he probably voiced the opinion of many others who were not quite so outspoken. I was very pleased when he told me, after I had worked solidly for one year without ever calling in sick, that he was "pleasantly surprised at my behavior and work ethic." That conversation sparked other conversations, which led to a great camaraderie between us. Our positive interactions showed other colleagues that I had truly been "accepted" into the group. This acceptance led to many collaborations with other colleagues, which ultimately helped me progress from assistant professor to associate professor, and, most recently, to full professor.

I realized that, although they may not always look like you, supportive people can help you progress and possibly become role models. That is a key message that I would like to offer. We must elicit the assistance of the people who can help us, regardless of any differences. We need to find the people with whom we are friendly or with whom we have some sort of bond, but, most important, we must find those whom we want to emulate. We must talk with them and express to them the similarities we share so that in mentoring us they will focus on those similarities and not on what is different.

I enjoy my career, and I enjoy my family, but I cannot give 100 percent of me to them both simultaneously. I try to schedule time off from work so I can chaperone a field trip or participate in another activity with my children. I take time to attend their games and talk with their teachers. The time I spend with my family is limited but precious, so I make sure that the time is quality and golden. When there are extra demands at work, I spend more time in the office or in the operating room. To make deadlines, I push the date up to make sure that last-minute distractions do not become derailments. And, when I go home, I leave the office at the office. Finally, I forgive myself when things do not happen as I expect they should. I take my lemons and make lemonade.

Outwardly, some would say that I am successful. How do I define success? Booker T. Washington said it best: "Success is to be measured not so much by the position that one has reached in life as by the obstacles which he has overcome." I am sure that overcoming obstacles is not unique to African-Americans or to women. In fact, for me, striving to overcome obstacles has strengthened my character and resolve. When I fall, I pick myself up and dust myself off, for as Maya Angelou says, "I am the dream and the hope of the slave. I rise, I rise, I rise."

Mae Jemison, the first female African-American astronaut, dared to dream of flying into space even when she did not see any other astronauts who were African-American women. Oprah Winfrey dared to become a media mogul by breaking new ground and creating "an unparalleled connection with people around the world." Shirley Jackson, the 18th president of Rensselaer Polytechnic Institute and, according to *Time* Magazine, "perhaps the ultimate role model for women in science," dared to dream of becoming a physicist. And Vivian Porche dared to become the first African-American female professor in M. D. Anderson's history. I believe the two things we all have in common (besides, of course, our ethnicity and gender) are our pursuit of excellence and our perseverance. With God's help, we can *all* achieve our most lofty dreams.

Kristen J. Price, M.D.

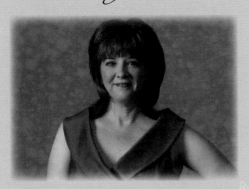

Professor and Chair of Critical Care

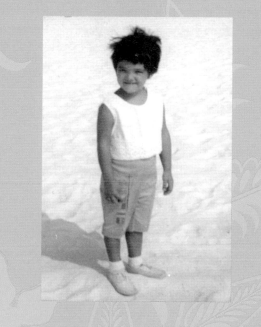

Kristen's fascination with nature and science began about age 4 when she played on the beaches along the Florida Gulf Coast.

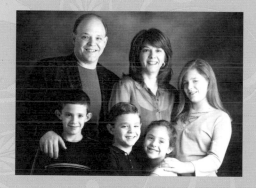

Husband Eric Price and Kristen with children, from left, Eric, Ryan, Claire and Elise.

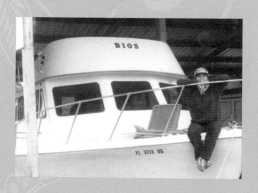

Kristen has many memories of Bios, the University of Tampa's marine science research boat.

I was born the fifth of six children in New Orleans, Louisiana. Some of my earliest childhood memories are of those exotic vacations our family took to the Mississippi or Alabama Gulf Coast. If we were really lucky, we would actually get to load up the station wagon and drive to Pensacola, Florida. What I remember most about those vacations is not building sand castles or eating in the elaborate dining room of the Holiday Inn. Instead, what I remember best is being awestruck by the power and beauty of the waves hitting the shore. I realize now that the Gulf Coast is a bit shy of an island paradise, but to me it was just about as close to heaven as a 5-year-old kid could get! I would watch the waves for hours on end, and I now know that it was that innocent amazement regarding nature that sparked my love of science and, ultimately, led me to a career in clinical academic medicine. As with most of life's journeys, there have been many twists and turns along the way. Some have been difficult, some most wonderful, and all have been amazing. What follows is my story, and I hope some insight into what I consider the privilege of being a daughter, wife, mother, physician and administrator.

I am not sure whether it was birth order or genetics, but I was a very independent, self-sufficient child. I can remember thinking as a very young child that it was important for me to do something good with my life, and I can remember worrying that I needed to be perfect. I loved the idea of going to school, so you can imagine the agony I suffered at age 5 when we moved to a neighborhood where the Catholic school did not have a kindergarten! My mother had already taught me to read, so I spent most of that year reading anything and everything in the public library. By the time I finally was able to start school, I had become enamored with marine biology and set out on a quest to become the first "female Jacques Cousteau." That previous year in the library had paid off, as I had been fortunate to stumble upon a series of books that Cousteau had written on marine science and oceanography. I read them all!

As is the case with most children, family events in those early years helped shape my views and motivations. My mother was ever supportive, especially as she had been born to Italian immigrants who did not believe in higher education for women. I listened intently to her stories about her childhood dreams of becoming a physician — dreams that unfortunately were not supported by her parents. What a phenomenal physician my mother would have been! She was the neighborhood medic and the "go-to" mom for cuts, scrapes, impaled objects and other minor emergencies. Her influence on my life is indescribable on so many levels, and I truly believe that watching her selfless actions ultimately led me to choose a career in medicine over marine science. My father, on the other hand, influenced me in a much different way. He divorced my mother when I was 10 years old and my younger brother was only 5. Now, nearly 20 years after his death, I ponder how a man could leave his family, and I still don't have an answer. Divorce affects children in many different ways. For a child like me, it was a heavy burden. I watched my mother struggle to single-handedly raise six children, and I felt helpless and anxious. I saw my role as "the perfect child." I was a straight-A student, the family peacemaker and the fierce protector of my younger brother, whom I believe suffered the most from my father's leaving. And so I progressed in this manner as I grew up, highly motivated and driven. I now believe that my father's actions intensified my need to lead a purposeful life and my drive for perfection.

In keeping with my quest to be "Jacqueline" Cousteau, I researched every marine biology program in the country — before I started high school! This ultimately led to four amazing years at the University of Tampa with degrees in marine science, biology and chemistry. I had a wonderful mentor there, Dr. Richard Gude. He built the university's research boat, the Bios (which our class got to name), and we had special "intersession" classes on that boat for a month at a time each year. It was truly an amazing experience. However, I began to have serious thoughts about becoming a doctor in my sophomore year of college. I did a lot of volunteer work then with the Catholic youth group, and found that I derived great satisfaction from helping people. So I completed the Marine Science program in Tampa but then returned to New Orleans to attend Louisiana State University School of Medicine.

Those next four years were quite different from school on the Bios, but my experiences as a medical student at Charity Hospital were incredible! During that time, I also met my husband (now of 23 years), Earl Mangin. In our senior year of medical school, we married, graduated and moved to Houston to do residency and fellowship training — all within a four-month period. On the first day of my internship, I was assigned to M. D. Anderson Cancer Center, and I was scared to death! However, I quickly learned what a phenomenal place it truly is, and I enjoyed every rotation I had here. After three years in an internal medicine residency, one year as chief medical resident, and three years in a pulmonary and critical care fellowship, I was hired as an assistant professor at M. D. Anderson. And so began my career in academic medicine. Earl completed his training in interventional cardiology and joined a private practice group at that same time.

We did not have family in Houston, and we had put having children on hold during our training. But six weeks after I joined the M. D. Anderson faculty, my daughter Elise was born. Six months after that, I became the medical director of the Medical Intensive Care Unit. Our son Eric was born two years later, followed by our daughter Claire two years after that. One of the beautiful things about bringing children into the world is that such an event forces you to reflect internally on your life. I had been the person who never had a task too big to accomplish. Now, my highly organized "superwoman" lifestyle was definitely becoming a challenge, and for the first time I felt that I couldn't do it all. The anxiety I had over that revelation was more than anything I had experienced throughout all my childhood! When I returned to work after maternity leave, I cut back my hours to 75 percent time, but that schedule was not easy to sustain in the department I was in at the time.

Then, as often happens, an unexpected event occurred when Claire was 3 months old. All three children came down with chicken pox, which would have been manageable if I hadn't been feeling so nauseated and fatigued in the morning. (I think you know where I am going with this!) Indeed, I was unexpectedly pregnant with our son Ryan. Obviously, infertility was never an issue for us! How many times do you think I was asked, "You're pregnant *again?*" Or, my personal favorite, "Two doctors and you don't know how to prevent that from happening?" As I reflect on those comments now, I think how sad it is that my own colleagues would be so overtly negative. I think the comments also struck me as negative then because I was still so conflicted over my drive to continue to run the intensive care unit (even at a reduced time commitment) *and* my desire to be with my children more. After much personal reflection, and for the first time in my life, I allowed myself to realize that some of my drive to be perfect stemmed from my childhood experiences and that it was O.K. to be honest about it. Still, I struggled.

Then, in another one of life's little twists of fate, I met my most influential mentor, Dr. Thomas Feeley. He had just been recruited to M. D. Anderson from Stanford University to become the division head of Anesthesiology and Critical Care. One of his main initiatives was to integrate all of the adult Critical Care Services and oversee the construction of a 52-bed combined Medical/Surgical Intensive Care Unit. From the first meeting I had with him, I recognized how supportive he was of women faculty. He shared stories with me of how his colleagues at Stanford supported him when he was raising his children. He understood the conflict of being dedicated to both one's career *and* one's family. Not only did he support my working part-time, but he also recruited me into his division and provided me with back-up coverage so that I could reduce my hours. I remember him telling me, "It may not seem like it now, but your kids will grow up quickly, and you will work full-time again before you know it." I thought, "Are you kidding me? I have four kids under the age of 7!" But Dr. Feeley was very successful in recruiting additional intensivists to manage the clinical load in the new ICU. So, for the next three years I worked two to three days per week doing clinical research and running the respiratory care services.

Just as Dr. Feeley predicted, my children got older and entered school, and I gradually began to increase my hours again. I first took on a more active administrative role when I accepted the position of deputy chair of the Department of Critical Care. Although I had given up the majority of my clinical practice, I found a new niche in administration and was surprised at how much I enjoyed it. Organization and time management were always strong points for me, so I was able to help my department chair expand our clinical, administrative and academic services. And since problem solving and conflict resolution are major means of survival when you grow up with five siblings and then parent four children of your own, I found that I was well suited to the job.

Three years ago, the position of chair of the department became available. Dr. Feeley and others encouraged me to apply, but I was torn once again. I knew I could run the Critical Care department well, but I suspected that some members of the search committee (made up almost exclusively of male colleagues) would raise a collective eyebrow. Indeed, when I walked into the panel interview, the first words a senior male faculty member said to me were, "You're right on time. It must be because you are the mother of four children and have to be organized!" Undaunted, I proceeded with the interview, answered all of their questions (including the not-so-subtle ones hinting about my previous part-time schedule and having children), and outlined my five-year strategic plan for the department. Needless to say, I got the job, and with Dr. Feeley's support, I was promoted to full professor in 2005.

Now, as I enter my fourth year as chair, I am proud to say that Critical Care at M. D. Anderson has grown to a group of 10 outstanding faculty members dedicated to providing evidence-based clinical care for the most critically ill patients in the institution. Our department also includes nine mid-level providers and 11 administrative staff. We are currently developing a research infrastructure that will encompass basic, translational and clinical research. Although we recognize that we will never cure cancer directly, we are committed to partnering with our oncologic colleagues to improve outcomes in the Intensive Care Unit. I developed the "Intensive Care Unit Organizational Infrastructure" to systematically organize, establish and sustain evidence-based clinical, educational and research initiatives in the Intensive Care Unit. This model comprises 10 specialized committees, each charged with developing, planning and implementing processes in their specialty area. Each committee is chaired by a member of the Critical Care faculty, is co-chaired by a member of ICU nursing leadership and has members from the key multidisciplinary services who provide care in the ICU. The Best Practice Committee, which I chair, coordinates all committee initiatives that enhance best and safe patient care. This model, described in detail on our department Internet site, has scored tremendous accomplishments in the past year. Numerous projects have flowed successfully through the infrastructure, resulting in improved patient safety. I am proud of this committee because it allows all ICU disciplines to work together for the benefit of our critically ill cancer patients.

And so, from wide-eyed little girl on the beach in Florida to wife and mother of four to department chair of Critical Care at M. D. Anderson Cancer Center, I conclude this portion of my story and look forward to the chapters to come. I am, quite frankly, one of the most fortunate women alive. I am deeply grateful to my mother, who has been my role model for my entire life, to my husband and children, who inspire me and have taught me to not take the world (and myself!) quite so seriously, to the amazing patients of this cancer center, who are an endless source of inspiration to me every day, and to Dr. Thomas Feeley, who is the type of mentor I wish every woman could have. My life and my career are rewarding beyond anything I ever could have imagined, and it is my sincere hope that I can serve as a role model for other women, especially those pursuing a career in academic medicine here at M. D. Anderson.

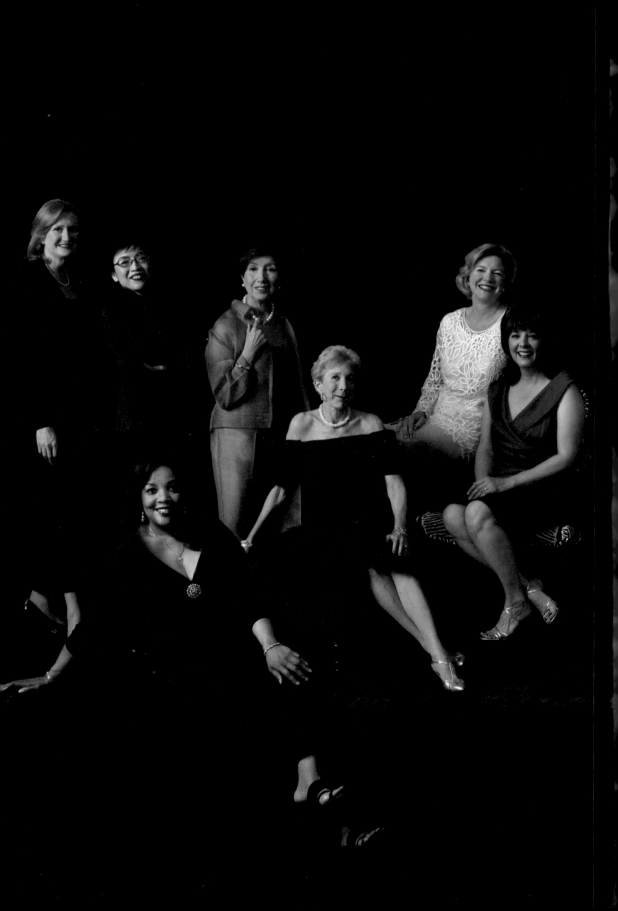

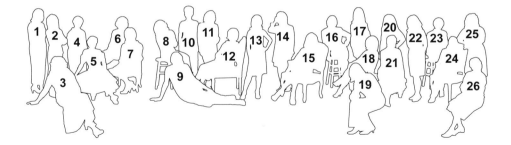

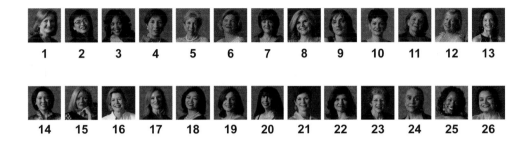

1   Sharon Y. R. Dent, Ph.D.
2   Dihua Yu, M.D., Ph.D.
3   Vickie R. Shannon, M.D.
4   Margaret R. Spitz, M.D.
5   Ellen R. Gritz, Ph.D.
6   Cheryl L. Walker, Ph.D.
7   Kristen J. Price, M.D.
8   Elizabeth Shpall, M.D.
9   Funda Meric-Bernstam, M.D.
10 Guillermina Lozano, Ph.D.
11 S. Eva Singletary, M.D.
12 Margaret L. Kripke, Ph.D.
13 Eugenie S. Kleinerman, M.D.

14 Karen H. Lu, M.D.
15 Elizabeth L. Travis, Ph.D.
16 Louise Connally Strong, M.D.
17 Kelly K. Hunt, M.D.
18 Ritsuko Komaki, M.D.
19 Elizabeth A. Grimm, Ph.D.
20 Razelle Kurzrock, M.D.
21 Peggy T. Tinkey, D.V.M.
22 Carmen P. Escalante, M.D.
23 Janet M. Bruner, M.D.
24 M. Alma Rodriguez, M.D.
25 Vivian H. Porche, M.D.
26 Varsha V. Gandhi, Ph.D.

M. Alma Rodriguez, M.D.

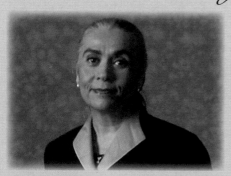

Vice President for Medical Affairs
Professor of Lymphoma and Myeloma

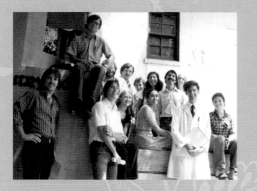

Alma, fourth from left, and other Class of 1979 students at The University of Texas Medical School at Houston are shown with Professor Henry Strobel.

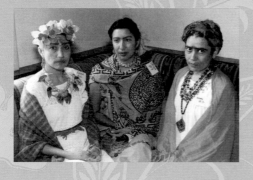

Two friends joined Alma, at right, in their imitation of painter Frida Kahlo, whose famous eyebrows intrigued the trio.

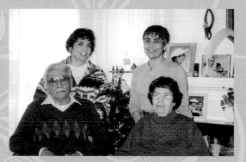

Alma, standing right, celebrated Christmas 1996 in San Antonio with her sister Oliva and their parents Ricardo and Oliva Rodriguez.

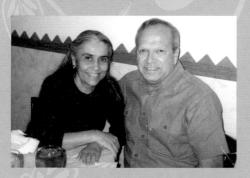

Alma and her partner Robert Trevino were happy to smile for the camera during dinner at a favorite restaurant in 2005.

am often asked how I chose medicine as a career and at what point I knew that I would become a physician. The most succinct answer is that it was a series of serendipitous events that led me to where I am today. I was born in Robstown, Texas, and raised in Roma, a small town on the U.S.-Mexico border in one of the poorest counties in Texas. My parents were migrant farm workers. Thus, the family was home (more or less) during the school year, but during the summer and early fall, we moved around doing seasonal farm work. I'd be willing to bet that the way my life has turned out definitely contrasts with most sociological predictive models!

It was in high school that I first discovered that I liked science. My best "aha!" moment occurred the day we learned about the Table of Elements, and I saw in a flash how Mandeleev's arrangement was brilliant and simple at the same time. I liked the order, simplicity and beauty of the elements and their atoms, and I hoped that one day I would become a chemist. However, in my family's history, no one had ever attended college, and although I was encouraged by my teachers to aspire to get a higher education, my family did not have the financial resources. There was no way I could get a higher education without scholarship support, and I had no clue of how to go about applying for it.

Fortunately, in my senior year of high school I was offered a full-tuition scholarship to Our Lady of the Lake University (OLLU), a small Catholic liberal arts college in San Antonio to which I had applied only because of encouragement from a neighbor whose daughter had attended the school. I accepted the scholarship, and, in the end, this chance event provided me with a wonderful opportunity. Classes were small, the professors knew each student by name, and every student was assigned a mentor, usually in their field of interest. Furthermore, most of the professors were women, who served as role models and inspired confidence that women could achieve academic success. This was a distinctly different experience, I learned later, from the experiences of my friends who attended larger state universities.

My initial mentor was Dr. Antonio Rigual, a Spanish literature professor who was passionate about Hispanics becoming more represented in all fields of academia, and I credit him for inspiring in me a sense of responsibility to lead and to open paths for future generations of students. In my freshman year, I took many science courses and did well, so Dr. Rigual encouraged me to declare a science major and to consider a career in the health professions. However, Mandeleev's esthetically ordered vision of matter — ranging from the subatomic to the molecular to the galactic — was very appealing to me, and so chemistry became my favorite discipline of study. Sisters Jane Slater and Isabel Ball were my mentors in the science majors program, and they encouraged me to pursue a graduate education.

Through an unexpected route, my study of chemistry actually led me to medicine. In my junior year, while I was contemplating applying to a graduate chemistry program, a second serendipitous event occurred. Two medical students from Baylor University came to the OLLU campus to recruit students of ethnic minorities for a special summer program. I applied to the program because it required a laboratory preceptorship in any one of several disciplines, including biochemistry, and I wanted to get biochemistry laboratory project experience on my resume to strengthen my application for graduate school. The catch was that we also had to attend classes and symposia aimed at preparing us to apply to medical school, but I figured that the laboratory experience I gained would offset the inconvenience of the classes.

My co-participants and I were grilled and drilled daily on academic questions and subjects that apparently were important to passing the MCAT, the medical school entrance exam, which I'd never heard of. The program also integrated exposure to clinical activities, including visits to an ER, where we saw gunshot victims wheeled straight into the OR; to an anatomy class, where we observed medical students performing dissections; to the observation galleries over the surgery suites at prominent hospitals, where we saw heart bypass procedures; and to labor and delivery, where we saw babies born. My lab project of isolating isoenzymes of a kinase from the regenerating limbs of salamanders was very interesting, but having seen all these aspects of medicine in real time convinced me, by the end of that summer, that I should apply to medical school.

That was 30 years ago, and since then it's been a most interesting adventure. I am not sure exactly when oncology became my destined discipline, but it probably started (at least subconsciously) with the first patient I ever examined as a medical student at The University of Texas Medical School on physical examination rotation at M. D. Anderson Cancer Center. The patient, a young man with congenital defects that included learning disabilities, had a malignancy that had brought him to M. D. Anderson. His mother agreed to my examining him on the conditions that she be present and that I not bring up the subject of his cancer, as she was trying to shelter him from this knowledge. I started with the usual textbook question, "What brought you to the hospital?" and he answered, clearly and distinctly, "I have cancer." That day, I learned a very important lesson, one that is almost universally true: if we ask the right questions and then listen, patients tell us what is wrong. This was a landmark day not only for me but also for the patient's mother. I still remember that young man's name, and it turned out that he had lymphoma. That was perhaps a prophetic encounter, since the treatment of cancer — and specifically lymphoma — ultimately became the focus of my career.

When I finished medical school, however, I thought that my path was to become a general internist and work within the Hispanic community where, unfortunately, diabetes, hypertension, and cardiac illnesses are rampant. Thus, I applied for a residency at The University of Texas Medical School affiliated hospitals in San Antonio so I could get good experience in treating these conditions. However, it turned out that the most engaging and interesting teachers and patients were in the Oncology Service. The attending physician, who became my mentor, was Dr. Daniel Von Hoff, a young and enthusiastic oncologist who was a tireless dynamo and advocate of new drug development. He also advocated personalized drug treatment based on each individual patient's tumor-sensitivity assays. Dan's dream of individualized treatment directed by personalized assays has finally reached the mainstream of oncology research, and it may in the near future come to fruition in the clinical setting. Through Dan, I learned of the drug development program at the University of Arizona's Cancer Center, which led to my fellowship training there. Again through serendipity, upon finishing my fellowship, I found that one of the oncologists in Arizona knew of an open position in the Lymphoma section of the Hematology department at M. D. Anderson. It was thus that I came full circle 20 years ago, returning to the hospital where I had had my first patient encounter.

I started my career at M. D. Anderson as a laboratory researcher and a clinician. During my fellowship, I had spent two years in the laboratory of Dr. Brian Durie working with lymphoid and myeloma cell lines, and I thought I would continue this path in laboratory investigation. Over the span of my first six years at M. D. Anderson, however, I lived like a nomad, frequently moving my projects from one lab to another as my bench space changed locations. It was also a difficult time of leadership transition in the Department of Hematology. During this time, the department had at least three chairpersons and, ultimately, it was restructured into three separate departments. I realized one day, after yet another failed grant application and while packing my bench in anticipation of yet another pending laboratory space change, that to succeed as a serious basic science investigator would require far more focus, direction, time and concrete infrastructure support than I had. This was a point of identity crisis for me, and I felt that I had to choose — the bench or the bedside. After all the years I'd spent honing my skills as a clinician, I knew that the clinical aspect of my work was very precious to me, and I did not want to give it up. So, I chose to focus my career on clinical work and said goodbye to the laboratory. Several of my colleagues declared that my choice was foolish, as I'd already devoted so much time to laboratory investigation. I, however, thereafter gained a greater sense of stability in my life and decided to focus on and make the best of the path I'd chosen.

In a recent interview, I was asked if I had a favorite or inspiring quote that I treasured, and indeed I do. It's a statement I read long ago, wrote down in one of my journals, and have made one of my life's guiding principles: "Don't let what you can't do keep you from doing what you can." That is my pragmatic approach to adversity and change: if life or circumstances block a path in your life, simply look in another direction. There are 360 degrees of spatial rotation around us, and somewhere in that circumference, there'll be a new way to go.

In my career at M. D. Anderson, I have been most fortunate to have the support of excellent mentors. Dr. Lillian Fuller was a very important mentor in my development as a clinical investigator. She was a professor of radiation oncology, with a focus on the treatment of lymphomas. She had joined the faculty of M. D. Anderson when Dr. R. Lee Clark was the president and leader of the institution, and she had worked side by side with the visionaries who founded M. D. Anderson. Thus, her historical perspective was wise and inspiring. She encouraged me and invited me to develop projects with her. She was a very disciplined writer, and when I worked with her, she required that we devote hours to writing and revising papers. She had a very significant influence on my career. Dr. Fernando Cabanillas, chief of the Lymphoma section and later chair of the Lymphoma-Myeloma department, was also a supportive advocate. He provided research protocol opportunities for me to lead, encouraged me to travel and present at international meetings and conferences, and introduced me to leaders in the field of lymphoma therapy. Having his support and advocacy was critical for my professional development. The culture of the Lymphoma section when I joined it was one of collegial and respectful behavior, and I never felt left out or had my opinions disregarded in discussions or planning. I have been fortunate and have had wonderful colleagues in the Lymphoma department who have been and continue to be my collaborators and who have valued my collaboration in protocols; together we've done creative and productive work.

The 1990s witnessed development of the institution's multidisciplinary clinic concept, and clinics were reorganized with new clinical leadership and a restructured administration. During that period of transition and clinic reorganization, Dr. Cabanillas assigned me to be medical director of the Lymphoma Center. Again, I was fortunate, as I discovered that I could apply the same processes of project organization, planning and data analysis that I had applied in the laboratory to the analysis and planning of clinical operations, and, as a result, a new direction for my life emerged. I learned a whole different perspective of medicine: the perspective of the complex economics that fuel the engine of the institution, the perspective of medicine driven by external forces — from the patients' point of view, from regulatory agencies, from government and from the law. Because of my role as a medical director, I got to know the hospital's operations leaders, and that eventually led to my current role as Vice President for Medical Affairs. When Dr. Thomas Burke was asked to fill the role of CEO of the institution in an interim capacity, he asked me if I, in turn, would fill in for him in his previous charge of Medical Affairs. That unexpected but fortuitous request has taken me on yet another journey.

In my current role, I am learning that the profession of medicine is poised for a historic paradigm shift that I believe is as significant as the change that occurred at the turn of the 20th century, when the training of physicians changed from individual apprenticeships to a more scientific, academic and hospital-based environment. The application of scientific principles and discoveries to categorize and understand the biologic basis of illnesses became the bedrock of medical education, and research and medicine became inseparable partners. The emerging new paradigms are of a different scale but are equally significant.

The new world of the future of medicine scrutinizes the decision making of physicians under the criteria of competence, guidelines, outcomes, cost-effectiveness, quality and safety, in addition to confirmed or supportive scientific data. While it is still critical that we understand the biology and scientific explanations of illnesses, an equally important element of medical practice now is how we apply concepts, knowledge, and new technology and pharmacology. The method of practice itself is a critical factor for successful outcome. The emergence of antibiotic-resistant microorganisms, for example, brings this principle to mind. The outcomes of infections and the prevention of resistance depend on multiple events: the processes of antibiotic choice (guidelines for appropriate use), timing and duration of delivery (efficient and proficient pharmacy and nursing support), and routes of administration (pharmacology and technology). These factors have as much importance and influence on the outcome of the patient's illness as understanding the basic cell biology or biochemistry of the microorganisms has.

As new technologies are developed in response to new scientific findings, innovations relevant to specific diseases, issues of cost, justice in access, safety and competence must be considered, but now the appropriate *application* of these innovations is emerging as an issue as important as are the innovations themselves. In the practice of oncology, these concerns are paramount, as, for example, when new drugs are developed. The extraordinary costs of recent new pharmacologic agents limit their access by some patients, and indiscriminate use of these drugs for unproven indications increases the cost of coverage for all patients. These situations create not only major socioeconomic health care issues but also ethical and, in some cases, legal concerns.

Thus, I continue to find new paths, and my journey is far from over. I think I am learning as much now as I did in medical school, but I'm absorbing totally different content. As my knowledge continues to broaden, I feel that I am still in the process of becoming a physician.

Vickie R. Shannon, M.D.

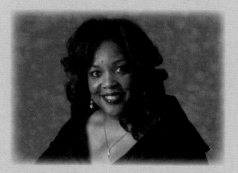

Professor of Pulmonary Medicine

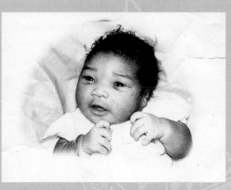

Vickie at three months

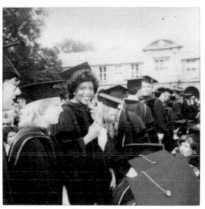

Vickie rejoiced with classmates when they graduated from Washington University Medical School in 1983.

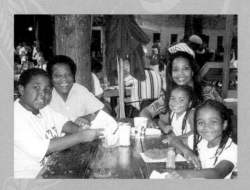

Her mother, second from left, and Vickie enjoyed lunch on the River Walk in San Antonio with Vickie's nephew Kamron and nieces Leanne and Bryanna.

y decision to become a physician was not fueled by any single pivotal event but rather by a series of unique circumstances, literally starting at birth, that has decisively underwritten my career choice and anchored my commitment to this profession. I was born in St. Louis, Missouri, at a time when St. Louis and the rest of the nation struggled with the prominent issues of race, racism, and the social upheavals of the civil rights movement and affirmative action. By the time I was born, the civil rights movement had already started to unravel some of the stiff racial inequalities that plagued this nation. Yet there were still rules, both tacit and overt, that dictated all forms of racial inequalities, from where blacks were born to where they were buried.

All of my older siblings had been born in the designated "black" hospital in St. Louis. Following the delivery of my older sister, something had gone terribly wrong. My mother lay in a pool of blood for hours, barely conscious, only yards away from the ignoring ears and eyes of the nursing staff. Several surgeries and several weeks passed before she finally emerged from that hospital, vowing to never go back there again. Two years later, with quiet determination and unruffled dignity, she rolled into Barnes Hospital, one of St. Louis' "white" hospitals, to deliver a 3.5-pound, premature baby girl she would name Vickie — me.

Sitting in the kitchen at age 14, I was mesmerized by Mother's recounting of the events leading to my birth. She spoke of her outrage following her near-death experience after the birth of my sister, not knowing at the time that this would be the necessary evil that would fuel her resolve to demand future health care elsewhere. She spoke of countless arguments with my father, who, fearing devastating consequences, insisted that she not "rock the boat." She recalled being nearly consumed with fear — which she veiled with stoic determination — as she entered the emergency room at Barnes, in labor after only 7 1/2 months of pregnancy, and how her emotions degraded to despair after sitting for more than 24 hours in the nearly empty waiting room after several failed attempts by the emergency room staff to redirect her and my father to the "black" hospital. Her eyes widened and voice quivered as she recalled the enormous amount of life-sustaining medical support and expertise that I required during my first few months of life — care that was at that time only available at Barnes — and how without these series of events, divinely timed and coordinated, my life would have been impossible.

What makes this story even more remarkable is an understanding of my mother's personality. Mother has always been a very soft-spoken, sweet-natured woman with an incurably demure personality. Although she witnessed many heinous acts of racism while growing up in the South, the anger and oppositional spirit just were not in her. No matter how right my siblings and I were or how passionately we articulated our position during skirmishes that occurred in and outside our home, she would never miss an opportunity to drill into us the values of tolerance, temperance, personal responsibility and deferred gratification. For me and my older (and more rebellious) siblings, who grew up in the 1960s, those values fostered personal decorum and protected us from the harsh social upheavals that defined that period.

I guess the notion of becoming a physician first occurred to me at Grandmother Ella's funeral. I was 11 years old. Ten days before she died, Grandmother had been rushed to the hospital for management of hypoglycemia. She was diabetic. Two days later, the family was called into her hospital room, and a tall, gaunt physician with a scraggly blonde beard and a vacant stare told us that Grandmother had died "of natural causes."

Grandmother was a cheerful, hardworking woman who was the gravitational pull in the family. Born into very meager beginnings, she and my grandfather learned to be extremely resourceful. They could stretch a dollar bill to 10 times its value. This resourcefulness, coupled with a climate of racism that denied blacks easy access to stores, fostered self-reliance. My grandparents used these stumbling blocks as their stepping-stones. Grandmother made all of their clothing; all food, including milk, cheese, vegetables, meats, poultry and fish, were products of their farm. Even the furniture was made from trees on the property. Their thriftiness paid off. By the time my grandparents were 40 years old, they were financially comfortable. Their only major indulgence was the purchase of an expansive acreage of farmland with majestic trees whose branches stretched over large clear lakes — Mother Nature's swing sets and diving boards. Every summer, all of the grandchildren converged on our grandparents' house for a boisterous two weeks of fun under the sultry Mississippi sky. Being a city girl, I found the freedom inherent in rural living to be unmatched. It was better than going to Disney World. Years later, reminiscing with my cousins about the "good old times" in Mississippi, we were all struck by the amount of discipline and hard work my grandparents maintained to keep a farm of that magnitude running smoothly and by how they insisted on managing the farm themselves, even though they by then had the financial wherewithal to hire outside help. Even more remarkable was their ability, through sweat, pluck and brains, to rise above the circumstances of their birth and the discriminating hands of larger society.

Standing at my grandmother's gravesite, overwrought with grief, I was struck by the sheer number of people in attendance — elderly couples, young families, single women with children, children who had come alone. All had come to pay their respects to the diminutive, gray-haired woman who had somehow affected their lives. They spoke of her unyielding spirit and her charity — not in the sense of pity or simple handouts, but as something more committed, more demanding. They spoke of her home as a welcoming source of refuge for the homeless, the sick and the frail. And they spoke of her indelible inner strength, buttressed by a fundamental faith in God, and of how that faith sustained her during the loss of her husband and several children. I walked away from the gravesite not depressed, but inspired, knowing that her legacy of charity and benevolence would somehow survive through me. I had always held a certain fascination with the sciences and had done well in these subjects in school. Melding my love for the sciences with my desire to carry on Grandmother's legacy of charity through a career in medicine just made sense. Grandmother's death may have *inspired my desire* to become a doctor, but it was her immortal teachings of perseverance, drive, discipline and charity that would *sustain my interest* in medicine through the years.

I was a junior at Smith College in Northampton, Massachusetts, pondering choices for medical school. Should I stay on the East Coast? Cover new ground on the West Coast? Go back to St. Louis or other parts of the Midwest? Then, it finally hit me with undeniable clarity: I would enroll in Washington University School of Medicine. That university's teaching hospital was Barnes Hospital. The irony of it all was almost laughable: I would return to the institution that had nearly rejected me at birth. The physicians who were willing to foreclose on my life 20 years earlier would now become my mentors, teaching me how to heal others. My life had come full circle.

During my senior year at Smith, my brother died. Stanley, a policeman and father of three, was murdered while on duty. His death blanketed the family with silent, unspeakable agony. In the weeks and months that followed, I immersed myself in academic and volunteer work. One of the most memorable places where I volunteered was at a homeless shelter for battered women and their children. I was hired as a junior counselor. To this day, I do not know what inspired me to work at that facility or how I even found the place. It was a small facility, strategically nestled in wooded hills in a remote area outside Northampton. My sheltered *"Leave it to Beaver"* upbringing had not exposed me to or prepared me for any of the assaults and losses these women and children had experienced. In the weekly counseling sessions, the women spoke of horrendous losses: their homes, livelihood, and for some, even their health and children had been destroyed. No matter how painful their stories were, however, not once did I hear bitterness or a sense of vengeance in their voices. A recurring theme that emerged from many of these sessions was their faith in God — but not faith as I had known it. Having attended a Baptist church while growing up, I understood faith as an abstract entity that one called upon to circumvent death or comfort the weary. In the final hours of my brother's life, I was angry that my prayers and faith had not changed his outcome. For these women, however, faith was something that was unconditional and, therefore, more enduring, more tangible. They lived out their faith, understanding that their relationship with God was not conditioned by having Him submit to their will but rather by their submitting to His will. By the end of my senior year, I was sorry to leave. I may have been hired as their counselor, but the people at that shelter taught me so much. Although I learned a lot at Smith, some of my most precious lessons were discovered outside the classroom.

I took these indelible lessons with me as I matriculated to medical school at Washington University, and they have helped guide me throughout my life. One of the mistakes that I made early on at Washington University was not finding a mentor. Attribute it to the filtered values of self-reliance from my grandmother or to my mother's teachings of discipline and personal responsibility; I wrongly thought that mentorship was a waste of time. I was busy attending class, tutoring underclassmen, volunteering at my church and a local nursing home, and playing tennis. Sitting with a mentor, I thought, would only add to an already overburdened week. In retrospect, I realize that I was wrong. A good mentor can be a valuable lifeline, offering assistance with issues ranging from academics to eateries. A good mentor would have suggested that I not overburden myself (as I did) with too many extracurricular activities during the earliest stages of my training. Certainly, a mixture of academics and extracurricular activities is healthy, but crafting a balance between the two is something that a more seasoned person who had gone through a similar experience might have been particularly helpful in facilitating. Even more important than having smarts and knowing where to find the best pizza parlor, a good mentor must have several durable, but frequently elusive, attributes: authenticity, honesty and empathy. These qualities distinguish mentors as leaders and true mentorship as a mission rather than a business. As time passes, I find myself looking for and appreciating these qualities more and more, internalizing and integrating them into my own moral code.

Towards the end of my medical school training, I began to wrestle with choices for internship and residency training. I had boiled it down to two areas: obstetrics/gynecology and internal medicine. I loved assisting with deliveries during my obstetrics rotations but also found the more cerebral aspects of internal medicine appealing. Finally, I decided to apply for an internship and residency in internal medicine, thinking that the thrill of delivering babies at 2 a.m. might eventually wane. My choice was a good one. Upon completion of my residency training, I accepted an offer for fellowship training in pulmonary and critical care medicine at my alma mater, Washington University. There, I met Dr. Michael Holtzman, chief of Pulmonary Medicine at that time and a brilliant scientist and mentor. I worked in his research lab for two years during my fellowship, studying the role of arachidonate products in the development of airway inflammation. Although I found the research exciting and even published original articles in scientific journals under his tutelage, bench research was for me too incremental and too far removed from direct patient care. Around this time, I was also growing tired of St. Louis. I knew that I wanted to remain on staff at an academic center, but I desired to venture into other parts of the country.

I must admit that I came to M. D. Anderson Cancer Center on a whim. I had been invited for an interview and came for what I thought would be a quick weekend. More than a decade later, I am still here. I take pride in the work I do here and the contributions I make to patient care, teaching, and clinical research. I enjoy the academic environment here, which is bustling with students, residents, fellows and colleagues who are intelligent, curious, intense, critical, anxious and excited. These qualities magnify the many challenges of teaching, a role that I thoroughly enjoy. Most of all, I love my work as a clinician. Often, the pace is frenetic, and the days are long and unpredictable. This type of schedule is embedded in a career in pulmonary and critical care medicine. It comes with the territory. That's O.K. — as long as I know that, at the end of the day, my work has positively affected my patients' lives. Making a difference in these patients' lives while they maintain hope and dignity in the direst of circumstances has been a personally rewarding experience for me.

Last year, for the first time in the history of M. D. Anderson, two African-American women were promoted to the rank of full professor. I was one of them. The immediate reaction of many of my colleagues (after offering their congratulations) was "Why did it take so long for a black woman to be promoted to this position?" For this question, I have no rightful answer. I do believe that, as in other aspects of achievement among blacks, what deserves focus is not the number of blacks that failed to succeed but rather those who succeeded against all odds. The promotion is a milestone for me as well as for M. D. Anderson and is a reward for my hard work and accomplishments in and outside of the hospital.

My work in hospital and community-based volunteer programs has grown out of a need to give back to a larger community in a world in which such basic needs as food, clothing, housing, education and health care are distributed unevenly. Career Mentors, a program for impoverished, inner-city elementary school systems, is one such program to which I have devoted my time almost since first arriving in Houston. This initiative allows students to regularly interact on a one-on-one basis with a diverse group of professionals, including lawyers, physicians, nurses and businesspersons. Such networking opportunities have proved invaluable to these students, touching their lives well outside the classroom. I am also a long-term volunteer for the King Foundation preceptorship program, a summer program at M. D. Anderson for bright high school students in the Houston area. I have enjoyed working with these students and have found their research projects interesting. Students who have completed the program under my preceptorship have gone on to such schools as Duke, Harvard and Johns Hopkins and continue to excel academically. After completing the program, many of these students not only have considered career paths as physicians but as physicians in academic medicine. Those kinds of declarations come at a remarkable time, when uncertainties in funding, salary differentials and debt threaten the growth of the medical field. I am not sure when I transitioned from being a mentee to a mentor. Hopefully, through my leadership and advice, I can help students seeking mentorship avoid some of the gratuitous mistakes I made during that period of my training.

I grew up in a large, traditional family. Mother's charitable arms, a quality that she no doubt got from her mother, made our family appear even larger. I assumed during my childhood that my adult life would mirror that of my parents — that I would marry, have a career, have children and live happily ever after. And I am blessed with an exciting career that I love, but marriage and children have not materialized. As a single woman, I have stitched together a priceless network of friends and family that satisfies my need for meaningful relationships. My extended family includes adopted family members like Iliasu, a precious 5-year-old Nigerian boy whom I have sponsored for the past three years with money for food, clean water, clothing and education — items that many of us take for granted. I plan to meet him for the first time when I travel to Nigeria this summer. He's excited, and I am ecstatic about the prospect of our meeting.

Closer to home, I have helped take care of my brother Bryan and his young family. Although most of my family members have done well, rising tides do not lift all boats evenly. Bryan, a gifted musician with a promising career, developed heart failure following a heart attack at age 32. Suddenly, his life as he knew it was unrecognizable. With career derailed and a subsequent divorce, he became the custodial parent for his three small children, trying to make ends meet on a meager disability income. Although meeting the financial and spiritual needs of Bryan and his family while maintaining my own life here in Houston has been challenging, a larger challenge has been establishing boundaries that distinguish helpful assistance from disabling welfare. Striking this balance is important for Bryan to grow as a father and as a productive member of society. So, although I have no biological children, hopefully I have been a positive influence in many children's lives.

And marriage? Well, I'll just settle for two out of three for now.

Sometimes being a single physician is like winning the lottery. Distant relatives and long-lost friends come from near and far with suffocating demands on your time — *but only if you let them*. It is easy to tilt the scale too heavily towards work or to become consumed with other persons' issues if there is no immediate family to go home to. Whether it is weighing competing claims of work and family or work and other demands on your time, finding a balance between competing demands is imperative. Striking this balance is no less important for a single person. It requires setting boundaries and making personal time a priority. I was years into my career before I finally learned this lesson and was able to say "no" without feeling guilty. One way to free up time is to hire other people to do certain domestic jobs. This was another source of guilt for me. For example, at the start of my career I refused outside domestic help, thinking that as a single woman I should care for my home by myself. But the truth is, I don't know any woman — married or single — who after a 12-to-14-hour work day revels in the idea of going home and mopping her floors or cleaning her toilet.

I recall following my grandmother's funeral the conversation with my sister, Yolanda, when I announced to her my notion of becoming a doctor. "You should do what makes you happy," she said. Over the years, the sense of what makes me happy has become more clearly defined. As a physician and mentor, what makes me happy is the knowledge that, in some demonstrable way, I have been able to help people live their lives with some measure of dignity and that my career has allowed me to reach persons in my family and community that I would not have been able to reach otherwise. My advice to those at crossroads in their careers is to pursue what makes you happy. Pursue the career that would continue to hold your interest even if there were no monetary incentives. Find mentors and create a circle of support to help you as you develop your career, and hold on to the dream with dogged conviction. Use stumbling blocks as your stepping-stones.

Elizabeth Shpall, M.D.

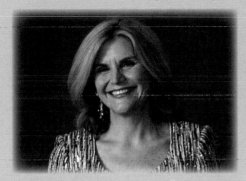

Professor of Stem Cell Transplantation and Cellular Therapy

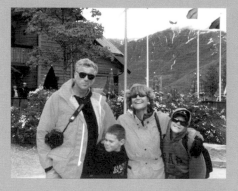

Elizabeth and husband Roy Jones, M.D., Ph.D., vacationed with sons Benjamin and Gregory in the Norweigian Fjords in 1997.

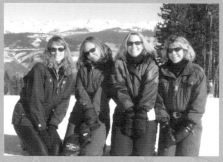

Skiing in Vail, Colorado, in December 2007 was great fun for this group, right to left, Elizabeth, her sister-in-law Debbie Rosenthal, sister Casey Shpall and sister Stephanie Shpall.

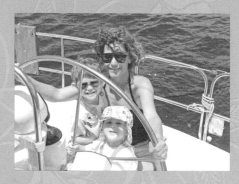

Sons Benjamin and Greg enjoyed sailing with Elizabeth in the British Virgin Islands in March 1993.

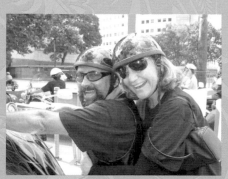

Daniel Minnehan, who had a stem cell transplant for leukemia in 2002, took his favorite physician, Elizabeth, on the Bad to the Bone Marrow Ride in 2007 to raise funds for transplantation research and recruit new stem cell donors.

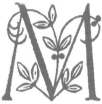y standard answer to the question "When did you decide to become a physician?" was "I always wanted to be a physician." But writing my story forced me to review all the stages of my life, and, after taking the time to reflect upon them, I came to realize that my usual answer was not quite true. My father was a physician — an extremely talented and empathic general practitioner who was loved by his patients and often cared for several generations in a single family. Some of his patients who had minimal financial resources paid him with produce from their gardens or with homemade jam. He delivered babies, performed minor surgeries, and was a gifted diagnostician. Growing up, I often went with him on house calls and Sunday morning hospital rounds and in doing so developed a profound and lasting admiration for his craft. Such was my early exposure to the medical profession. At the time, I did not consciously plan a career in medicine although, in retrospect, the subliminal attraction must have been there.

In my younger years, the things that were important to me were my horse and our happy family life in the bucolic foothills of Colorado. My parents had built their dream home on a mountain east of Golden and the Coors Brewery. A creative architect had designed it to look like a green and white shoebox sticking up out of the mountain. One side of the house was entirely glass with sliding doors that led out to a very large terrace. On clear days, which occurred frequently in Colorado, we could see the Snowy Range Mountains in Wyoming. Deer or red fox would often visit us, and we always felt like part of nature. My dad's friend, who sold horses, cattle and Indian jewelry, found me a gentle horse that was suitable for a 9-year-old. I named her Lady, and she could gallop as swiftly as the wind but was easy to control. Lady and I had many happy years together exploring the mountains around our neighborhood.

I recall with fondness the three wonderful years I spent in a serious academic program at rural Golden High School. As a freshman, I signed up for Latin and discovered a 70-year-old teacher who had refused to retire. The school board allowed her to continue teaching both Latin and classics. Since I was the only person who took her Latin course, I wound up having three years of private tutoring. I also had a great French teacher and again was lucky, as she taught the language and literature to only a handful of students for all three years. During this period, I came to realize that I would pursue some type of scholastic career, most likely in the area of arts and literature. My mother was from New York, and I decided that I wanted to study at a school on the east coast. The schools in that area that interested me the most were Harvard, Radcliffe and Brown. In the end I chose Brown because it had fine programs in classics in French and art history, two areas that I was particularly interested in. Moreover, Brown was known to be quite diverse and forward-thinking in terms of its curriculum as well as its student body, and I found the idea of exposure to that kind of atmosphere appealing.

When I initially arrived at Brown University, I majored in classics with a minor in French, and I dreamed of working for the State Department. My mother, an extremely intelligent, intellectual and independent thinker, very subtlety spoke of that period as being a time when women could be anything they wanted — Supreme Court justices, CEOs of major companies, physicians, scientists or architects, to name a few. My mother believed very deeply that women should pick difficult fields that they would enjoy and make contributions to the welfare of people everywhere. She was my greatest supporter and made me believe that I could really pursue and excel in whatever discipline I chose. Perhaps these ideas heightened my awareness of all the possibilities available to me. Then, during my first vacation from college, I noticed and was struck by how much my father still enjoyed practicing medicine. He studied a great deal, reading an enormous number of medical journals. In fact, he and I often discussed the medical issues he was interested in at the time. I guess that seeing him still retain his enthusiasm for medicine after all these years called up my childhood impressions of the practice of medicine and caused me finally to seriously consider it as a career.

When I returned to school in the fall, I took chemistry and biology courses to see whether I could handle them well enough to change my major to premed. This step set me on the path that would change the direction of my career and my life. I found that I liked the courses and did well in them. My studies at Brown gave me a great foundation for the challenging work that lay ahead. I loved the time I spent at Brown; those were wonderful years. Not only was I able to nurture my existing love of classics but also I discovered my love of biology while I was there. At Brown, I was fortunate to have a marvelous biology professor who truly instilled in me a love of science as well as a confidence in my scientific ability that I had never had before; for me, this truly opened the door to scientific inquiry. During these years, I spent several relaxing summers on the Cape with friends and even worked part time as a cocktail waitress. I think that these experiences helped round out my personality.

While I was in medical school and during my residency, I continued to expand my horizons intellectually, culturally and socially. I attended the University of Cincinnati College of Medicine and once again found that I had made a good choice. There, I was delighted to discover that I was part of a diverse, well-rounded and very talented class whose ranks included musicians and athletes, among others. Perhaps it was partly owing to the well-roundedness that stemmed from broad interests and talents, but, whatever the reason, there was among our class a wonderful espirit de corps. I loved medical school. The combination of interesting people, group camaraderie and stimulating courses was energizing. My interests tended more toward internal medicine type disciplines; I did not really care for anatomy or surgery courses very much. I had so much fun during this time and honestly remember these years as among the most enjoyable of my life. I spent my final year of residency taking electives at the American Hospital in Paris, where I lived in the hospital with medical students. To be studying abroad and in Paris was exciting and provided me with an enriching and fabulous experience culturally. I decided to do my subsequent training in New York City. I was not truly bitten by the research bug until my fellowship at the Mount Sinai Hospital, where I trained under the mentorship of Dr. James Holland, chairman of Neoplastic Diseases. Dr. Holland not only taught me an enormous amount but also instilled in me the confidence to pursue a career in academic medicine.

Dr. Holland also introduced me to Dr. Roy Jones, who subsequently became my husband and without whom I could never have become a public speaker! My husband and I were recruited to Duke University, where we had an academically rewarding experience working in the Bone Marrow Transplant Program with Dr. William Peters. The premier transplant program for breast cancer patients was at Duke, and this was our interest at that time. We welcomed our first son while we were working at Duke. We then went to the University of Colorado to establish a Bone Marrow Transplant Program. There we spent over a decade building the program and enjoying a rapid and productive expansion of our careers and our family, with the addition of our second son. I was fortunate enough to be able to establish a cord blood bank, which tied in with my clinical work in cord blood transplantation and laboratory work on the ex vivo expansion of hematopoietic progenitor cells with what became a major focus on expanding cord blood.

Subsequently, my husband and I were recruited to M. D. Anderson Cancer Center in 2002. It has been a marvelous move professionally, affording us academic and clinical opportunities in our field that are unparalleled, including a state-of-the-art Good Manufactory Practice Laboratory for cellular therapy and the establishment of another cord blood bank in Houston. While the move was exciting for us, our two sons, who had been avid hockey players and snow-boarders in Colorado since age 4, did not share our enthusiasm about moving to Houston, which occurred when they were in the 6th and 8th grades. As a consolation, we kept our place in the Colorado mountains, which allowed the boys to continue their winter sports during vacations. Although they have never really adjusted to the weather in Houston, they have attended great schools and made very good friends here. Our eldest son recently left to attend college at the University of Southern California Marshall School of Business in Los Angeles, and our youngest son, who will graduate from high school next year, will also likely choose a college outside of Texas. Fortunately, they still enjoy visiting with us, particularly when we are in Colorado.

My advice to women who are faced with the decision of whether to move the family for the sake of career advancement is to look at the big picture. If you will be happier and professionally more fulfilled, your family will ultimately benefit from your ensuing comfort and security. Now that my sons are leaving for college, it has become apparent that developing activities that you can do with your friends or husband is critically important. Tennis has always been my major outlet, but I have just started taking golf lessons as another option for the future. Although family and work have always been my main priorities, I recommend developing a hobby you enjoy in order to keep a balanced existence. In terms of career, my best advice is to focus. In academic medicine, pick an area you like — either clinical, laboratory, or, if you have the skills, both — and build upon it. Most large projects you take on should relate to your area of expertise. The more you develop depth in a discipline, the easier it is to be academically successful.

Academic medicine is a wonderful career. It is gratifying to be involved in cutting-edge therapies that may really improve the outcome in patients. Additionally, ascademic medicine involves highly collaborative and satisfying relationships with interesting colleagues around the world. Balancing the professional and personal aspects of one's life certainly presents challenges, but with focus and attention to your priorities, you can successfully blend the raising of children and a happy family life with professional success in the field of academic medicine.

S. Eva Singletary, M.D.

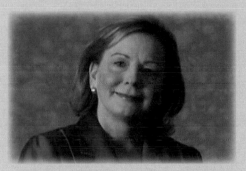

Professor of Surgical Oncology

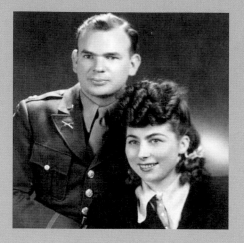

Eva's parents Joe and Agnes, whom he met during World War II.

(Photo courtesy of Springer Science and Business Media)

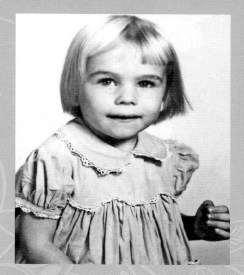

At age 3, Eva was already practicing the manual dexerity necessary to be a surgeon.

(Photo courtesy of Springer Science and Business Media)

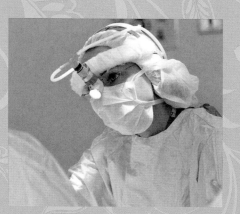

Eva schedules surgery for breast cancer patients most Tuesdays and Thursdays.

(Photo by F. Carter Smith)

ouston, Texas, where I have lived and practiced medicine for almost 25 years, could not be more different from the farm just outside of Coward, South Carolina, where I grew up. Although Coward was "town" when I was young, it was (and is) very small, not more than about three square miles, with around 600 people. Set in the lower watershed of the Pee Dee River in northeastern South Carolina, the country there is agricultural, producing crops of tobacco, cotton and soybeans. My father Joe returned there after serving in the European theater during World War II, but, rather than marrying the preacher's daughter as everyone had anticipated, he brought over and married Agnes, a stylish and refined woman he had met in Estonia.

Looking back, I am amazed and filled with admiration for how hard my mother worked to be a good farmer's wife and to contribute wherever she could. We had a small farm, growing tobacco and cotton as cash crops. Mother grew vegetables for us in a family garden. She also worked out in the fields, planting tobacco and picking cotton because it was a family farm and you did what was needed. She didn't let it bother her that people thought of her as a foreigner (at least at first) or that she had not really been raised for this kind of life. She got involved with the church, the 4-H club, the garden club — she was always ready to learn about something new, even if it wasn't in an ideal setting. I like to think of how valuable it was for her children to learn this important lesson early on.

There are things from those years that remain so vivid in my memory: seeing Mother with a kerchief on her head and a bucket in her hand, tending to the vegetable garden; assisting at my first "surgery" — an orchiectomy of a bull — at the age of 10; reading to my 4-H chickens to make them lay more eggs (an activity suggested by Mother). We were always encouraged — but not forced — to put ourselves out there and get involved, to not be afraid of competition, and to go after what we wanted, even if the circumstances were not ideal.

So, it was no surprise that when I was in junior high school and first announced that I wanted to be a doctor, I was met with encouragement from my parents, although they must have been gravely concerned about their daughter's venturing into a field where there were so few women. I was a good student, especially in science, so I don't think they ever doubted that I could succeed, and they were determined to give me the freedom to do what I wanted. They believed, and it proved to be true, that the things I had learned growing up on the farm — how to work hard, be well organized, never procrastinate and meet multiple deadlines — would be good tools for venturing into the world beyond.

When it was time for college, I chose Clemson University, located about

200 miles west of my home town. Clemson is a beautiful little college town with a lakefront setting against a backdrop of mountains and forests. It was originally part of the Cherokee Indian Nation, and you still see that influence in some of the geographic names: Issaqueena Falls, lakes Keowee and Jocasee, and Table Rock Mountain. The university was founded in 1893 by Thomas Green Clemson, a son-in-law of John C. Calhoun, South Carolina's favorite son. Thomas Clemson left his estate to be used to establish the school. At the time I was ready to enter college, Clemson University had just what I was looking for: a major emphasis in science taught in a small college atmosphere. Many of my classes had fewer than 20 students, so there was a lot of personal attention. It was exciting (and a little scary) being away from home for the first time, but I really had my eye on a more distant goal — medical school — so I devoted myself almost entirely to my studies and completed my bachelor's degree in a little over two years. Then it was time to engage the dream I had had since I was 12 and start the long, hard process of becoming a doctor.

The Medical University of South Carolina (MUSC) is located in Charleston, one of the oldest and most beautiful cities on the Atlantic seaboard. Home to one of the most active seaports in the world, Charleston is graced with huge oak trees and stately antebellum mansions. The College of Medicine at MUSC was the first medical school in the southern United States. When it opened in 1824 as a private institution, it had a faculty of seven Charleston physicians and 30 students. MUSC pioneered in clinical teaching, and its faculty members were responsible for some of the first medical textbooks in the United States.

I attended MUSC from 1977 to 1983. Early on, I made the decision to specialize in treating cancer patients. That meant going into surgery, since at that time, surgery was the only widely accepted treatment for many kinds of cancer. This was, I will admit, a little daunting: if there were *few women in medicine* at the time, there were almost *no women in surgery*. Surgical residencies were notoriously arduous, requiring a level of commitment that effectively ruled out having a normal life outside the hospital. Nonetheless, I was set on this goal. I figured that I had grown up on a farm and had already come this far, so a little more hard work wouldn't kill me.

My decision to become a surgeon was cemented during my last year of medical school, when students had the opportunity to rotate through the surgical services of several major medical centers. One of my rotations was at M. D. Anderson Hospital and Tumor Institute (as it was then named), where I had the privilege of meeting two individuals whose work was inspirational to an aspiring surgical oncologist. Dr. Richard Martin had just become chief of surgery at M. D. Anderson in 1977. He was one of four general surgeons, who did probably 95 percent of all the general surgical procedures performed at the hospital. Dr. Bob Hickey was an internationally known cancer surgeon. He was famous not only for his pioneering clinical research in endocrine tumors but also for his fierce advocacy at the national level for rehabilitation services to enhance the quality of life for cancer patients. These two role models demonstrated to me the innovative quality of the work that could be done in an academic environment and also impressed me with the teamwork philosophy that was to contribute to the development of multidisciplinary care at M. D. Anderson over the next 20 years. But, first, I needed to get through the difficult years of a surgical residency.

My surgical training took place at Shands Teaching Hospital, the primary teaching hospital for the University of Florida College of Medicine. Over the six years that I spent at Shands, I was well instructed in the technical aspects of surgery, but the most important things I learned came from being under the mentorship of Dr. Ted Copeland. Dr. Copeland was chair of the Department of Surgery at the University of Florida in Gainesville for 11 years, during which time that department became known as a rich and stimulating learning environment for residents and junior faculty. Although Dr. Copeland had an almost unbelievable list of academic achievements and honors, what impressed me was that he was a tireless advocate for his residents, students and fellows, something that I strive to emulate every day. He learned his surgical core values from the late Dr. Jonathan E. Rhoads at the University of Pennsylvania and passed them on to us: honesty; respect for patients, colleagues and trainees; education of the next generation; adding to the clinical and scientific knowledge base; not letting surgical decisions be income driven; and respect for tradition. He taught us to pay attention to the basics, to listen to our patients and be attentive to their comfort and safety, and to be prepared for the unexpected in the operating room. Finally, and perhaps most important, he taught us through the example of his own life how to achieve a balance between our lives as surgeons and our lives outside the hospital, allowing each to enrich the other. Recently, at the end of my term as president of the Society of Surgical Oncology, I selected Dr. Copeland as the recipient of the SSO Heritage Award, in honor of all that he has contributed to the field during his distinguished career.

I returned to M. D. Anderson in 1983 to undertake a two-year surgical oncology fellowship, after which I was invited to join the faculty as a general surgeon. I worked on a few research projects that used tissue culture models to answer some basic biological questions about tumor cells but didn't really feel that basic science was a good fit for me. I was more interested in clinical questions having to do with melanoma, and concentrated in that area for awhile, becoming chief of the melanoma section in the Department of General Surgery. But that focus changed when I met Dr. Eleanor Montague, who was then a professor of radiation oncology at M. D. Anderson.

Dr. Montague was an early advocate of breast preservation, pioneering the treatment of breast cancer using radiation therapy as an alternative to surgery. Because radical surgery had always been the treatment standard for breast cancer, the use of any breast-conserving therapy, let alone one that didn't even include surgery, was greeted as heresy by many. But as it turned out, clinicians like Dr. Montague started a movement toward less invasive treatment that continues to this day and has revolutionized cancer management. Dr. Montague was profoundly patient-oriented in her work and was a strong advocate of public health education and patient participation in treatment decisions. In addition, she was a wonderful mother to four children and always made them the central priority in her life. Dr. Montague was a major influence on my thinking with regard to my career and my life, and I redirected my emphasis into the study and treatment of patients with breast cancer.

The last part of the 20th century was an amazing and exciting time to be embarking on a career as a breast surgeon at a major cancer center. New treatments were being introduced every day, it seemed, and techniques that had been the cornerstone of breast cancer management for 100 years were being replaced. Standard treatment was becoming truly multidisciplinary, requiring input from radiation oncologists, medical oncologists, imaging specialists, plastic surgeons and pathologists. Patients with advanced disease, who 40 years earlier would have been dead within months, were now surviving much longer — sometimes for years. And advanced disease became much less common than before because more and more women were getting yearly mammograms, and the tumors being found were tiny and could often be treated with minimal surgery and radiation therapy. Staying up-to-date on the huge array of technical advances that had the potential to affect the treatment of breast cancer became almost a full-time job in itself, on top of the clinical work, research, teaching and mentoring that are part and parcel of a career in academic medicine.

Building a career in surgery involved overcoming numerous obstacles. Some were inherent to the field: meeting the physical requirements of numbingly hard work, juggling the multiple demands on my time, dealing with the grief and anger that arose on those occasions when I "failed" and a patient died. But some of the obstacles, trivial and not so trivial, stemmed specifically from being a woman in what has historically been an overwhelmingly male specialty. For example, until fairly recently, it was not uncommon for major institutions to have no separate dressing facilities for female surgeons, who were expected to share locker space with nurses. Many details about how academic medical departments were run (and are still run, in some cases) involved the expectation that clinicians would have no responsibilities or time commitments outside of their work. Critical meetings might be scheduled after normal working hours or on weekends, the promotion track was rigidly defined with no wiggle room to accommodate part-time work or leaves of absence, and schedules were assigned with no regard for the circumstances of parents with young children. There continues to be a tendency to replicate traditional gender roles in assignments meted out to junior faculty. Women physicians tend to be over-represented on department committees and are frequently involved in "co-authoring" (i.e., writing) book chapters or review articles at the request of senior colleagues. When I was a new junior faculty member, I remember being asked to serve on a committee involved with the inventory of surplus office furniture! I learned, with the aid of some wonderful mentors, to always stay focused on "what I was there for" and, accordingly, to avoid taking on commitments that were more associated with staff than with leadership. It is important for mentors to teach this to their mentees and to insulate them from the pressure to accept these tasks.

It has now been nearly 25 years since I came back to M. D. Anderson, and my priorities have evolved with the passing years. As a full professor, the "publish or perish" mentality aimed at promotion and tenure has become less important, so I can spend fewer hours involved with publishing clinical studies and with crisscrossing the country to attend endless professional meetings. I think it is important at this stage of my career to focus on those areas where I can really make a difference.

First, I focus on keeping abreast of technical advances in all fields that will help improve the treatment of my patients. In a century of multidisciplinary care, I believe that surgeons need to be at the forefront of coordinating that care for their patients. My writing has become increasingly channeled into comprehensive reviews that make these technical advances more accessible to other breast surgeons.

Second, I focus on mentoring fellows and junior faculty who are new to the field of surgical oncology. I know from my own experience that a strong mentor can make a critical difference to a young surgeon just beginning a career. In the words of my early mentor, Dr. Ted Copeland: "It is a unique privilege to serve as a role model for those who assume responsibility for the lives of others."

Third, I am passionately committed to patient education. I have always believed that to offer the best to my patients, I needed to be much more than just a good technical surgeon. Regardless of the stage of their disease, when women come to me for treatment, they are afraid, confused, unsure and sometimes angry. At first, they may not hear anything I say other then "cancer," and the visceral reaction they have to this terrifying word needs to be overcome with caring, thoughtful education. In addition to counseling my own patients, I have devoted considerable time and resources over the years to the development of educational materials for breast cancer patients, including pamphlets, books, videotapes, and most recently, interactive DVDs. The filmed materials provide new patients with the opportunity to "meet" women who have already undergone treatment and to learn how they handled the problems that arose along the way. The patients we have interviewed for these videos are nothing short of inspirational, and it is a privilege to be able to use their stories to help others.

I have saved the best and most important for last. My wisest role models over the course of my career always emphasized making your family a top priority. At one point, when my work was consuming my life, my mother said: "And let me remind you, young lady, that the walls of M. D. Anderson were standing before you got here, and they'll be standing after you leave. Don't think that you're the only one who can hold them up." That sage advice finally hit home with the birth of my son, Benjamin, the single most important person in my life. Watching him develop and grow and learn is an immeasurable joy every day. Sharing his experiences has given me new eyes through which to see the world and decide what is truly important. He has added a fresh focus that wonderfully informs and enriches both the personal and professional aspects of my life.

Margaret R. Spitz, M.D.

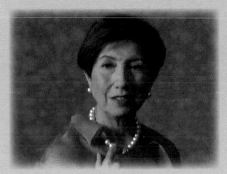

Professor and Chair of Epidemiology
Olga Keith Wiess Distinguished University Chair
for Cancer Research

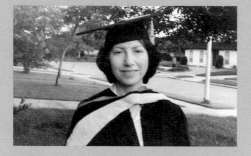

Margaret began her journey as an epidemiologist when she received a Master of Public Health degree from The University of Texas School of Public Health in 1981.

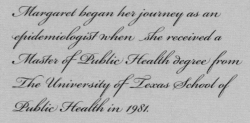

Drs. Joe Fraumeni, left, and David Schottenfeld congratulated Margaret when she received the 2003 Award for Research Excellence in Epidemiology or Prevention from the American Association for Cancer Research and the American Cancer Society.

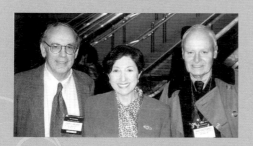

Margaret and husband Louis Berman, M.D., in 2005. At left, daughter Elise Berman Engels, M.D., and husband Eric Engels, M.D., with Joshua and Emma; in the center, son David Berman, M.D., Ph.D., and wife Sasha with Rebecca; right, son Howard Berman, Ph.D., with wife Randee and Sammy.

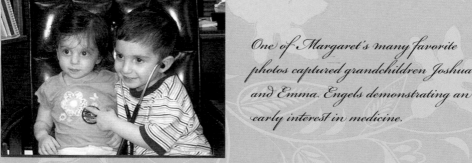

One of Margaret's many favorite photos captured grandchildren Joshua and Emma Engels demonstrating an early interest in medicine.

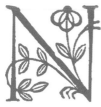owadays, my standard advice to young scientists or physicians is to "do as I say and not as I did." This is because some of the most momentous decisions I have made in my life seem to have been conceived on the spur of the moment. This is absolutely not an approach I advocate, but I have been lucky in that most of these knee-jerk reactions worked out remarkably well for me.

By nature I am not rash. In fact, as the youngest of three children, I was the most practical. Every Saturday morning my mother would drive us to the synagogue and give my brother (the oldest) the bus fare for our return home. My brother, who enjoyed the finest things that life offers, wanted to splurge the money on ice cream, and then we would have to walk home; my sister, the kindest of souls, argued to give the money to the barefoot little children who would congregate by the strip shopping center, and again we would have to walk home. I voted to use the money as intended — to catch the bus home — but I almost never won that argument.

The truth is that I never grew up wanting to be a physician. Rather, I was determined to be a nuclear physicist. As a child growing up in the privileged all-white enclave of Lower Houghton, in Johannesburg, South Africa, that seemed to me an exotic and challenging career and one that offered to bring me a little nearer to the unattainable land of my dreams, the United States of America. How could I have even guessed what my chosen profession entailed? The harsh reality was that I attended an all-girls high school that did not even offer us the choice of studying either physics or chemistry — those subjects were considered suitable professions *only* for boys. Girls were relegated to French and biology.

As an aside here, Joshua, my 8-year-old grandson, has a mother (my daughter) who is a radiologist. He already knows that he wants to be a doctor but when asked if he will read X-rays like his mother, his response is immediate and definite — "No, that is only for girls!!!" How times have changed in only one generation!

Returning to my story, my father was a wise man. Born in Lithuania, he escaped being drafted into the Russian army by crossing the border disguised as a girl, overcame "Jewish quotas" to be admitted to study medicine in Germany, and immigrated to South Africa in the early 1930s. His prescience about the future of the Jewish community in eastern Europe was supreme. Life experience taught him (and that became the overarching theme and mantra of our childhood) that as Jews, we could never consider ourselves to be safe and settled and that we must select "portable" professions in preparation for the time when we would again need to emigrate. It was not for me to question why nuclear physics was not considered to be in this category.

As graduation from high school neared, I was interviewed by the local newspaper and asked what I planned to study at The University of the Witwatersrand (Wits) in Johannesburg. Without thinking I blurted out "medicine." I had not even realized that I had already inexorably reached this decision. And thus was sealed my fate.

My first year at Wits Medical School was exceptionally challenging. I was one of a handful of women students and one who had never studied physics or chemistry. My days were miserable, and I barely made it through the first year. The next year, I was so uncertain about staying the course that my mother took me to a "guidance counselor," who advised me to "throw out your books and go get a bachelor's degree." I was outraged by this inane advice (and even more that my mother actually had to pay for it) and decided to carry on just to prove the counselor wrong. The Hebrew word for this attitude is "davka."

Things improved dramatically in the clinical years. Not that we as women weren't told consistently and often that we were taking the rightful place of men who needed the training to earn a living for their families and, moreover, that as women, we were destined to drop out and amount to little. For several, this in fact became a self-fulfilling prophecy. But not for me — I would prove them wrong. In the last two years of medical school, we were to form teams to rotate through various clinics. I was invited by some of the brightest and smartest of the male students to join their team, and we became known as the "A" team. Parenthetically, all but one now live in North America and one in Israel. The competition was fierce but manageable, and I seemed to thrive in this environment.

As graduation approached, we faced the prospect of choosing our internships. Dr. du Plessis, the professor of surgery at our medical school, was a brilliant surgeon but dictatorial and tyrannical. His internship was considered to be the pinnacle of prestige and highly sought after. One applied and he chose. He tolerated women in the operating room only if they were nurses. No woman had ever been selected as his intern. I doubt whether any had even had the temerity to apply.

I received a surprising phone call from his second-in-command, Dr. Bert Myburgh, asking me to formally apply for this honor. Without thinking twice, and knowing that this "honor" carried with it brutally long hours, a total absence of any hands-on experience, servile duties and prohibition of free expression, I unhesitatingly declined the "honor." There was a collective gasp of disbelief, and I was blackballed from all other surgical internships. There was no one to tell me that in all likelihood I had also dealt a setback to women's lib, and perhaps I had. This is also perhaps the reason why I am so in awe of the talented and dedicated women surgeons at M. D. Anderson today.

Marriage, three children and the decision to leave the land of our birth for America followed. This part of my story is in itself a long chapter, best left for another time, so I am flashing forward to the inexorable stream of events that led to our arrival in America.

A phone call from my physician-husband Louis Berman told me that he had taken a position as a rheumatologist at The University of Texas Medical School in Houston. First, the mad dash to a globe to locate Houston, as we knew only of Dallas at that time. Next, the trip to Austin to take the Boards, my 7-year-old daughter's school essay, "we are going to live in Texas, which is in Houston" (for which she received a perfect score), and the dreaded Visa Qualifying Exam. At first I was outraged when told that only one member of a family needed to pass the VQE. I wanted to earn this right to a visa on my own. And so my husband and I both sat for the English part of the exam, which was multiple choice. The questions were read by the wife of the American consul general, whom I later learned hailed from New Orleans and spoke with a very heavy Southern accent. I could not understand whether she was articulating "ankle" or "uncle" or "angle." As a result, I, who had always excelled at the King's English, almost failed the exam. I immediately decided to leave the science part of the VQE to my husband — another wise decision.

After arriving in Houston in 1979, I soon found it financially necessary to get a job and took a position as a physician in a home for the aged. I did not enjoy the way the American medical enterprise operated, so when a new director was appointed, and I found that I did not agree with his approach, I made a spot decision to resign. At this point, a friend suggested that I enroll in the UT School of Public Health.

A career in public health had never been a consideration. At medical school, our initiation into public health was through sewage farms that we were required to tour for credit. While I surveyed the optimal diameter for a latrine, the male students surveyed the cleavage of Dr. Erasmus, our voluptuous lecturer. If *this* was public health, I wanted no part of it. But eventually I did register at the UT School of Public Health, and I selected my classes based on their time slot, rather than on content, since I was then juggling priorities in order to supervise my three children, all under the age of 10. Car pools every day meant I could not take afternoon classes that ended after 2:30 p.m. This clearly was *not* the optimal way to learn epidemiology.

Initially, I was horrified at the casual atmosphere in the classroom: the way the students dressed, the freedom with which they brought drinks and food into the class, the impunity with which they challenged and argued with the lecturers and seemed to enjoy the interactions. This was definitely not what I was accustomed to. But gradually I learned to accommodate, and, two years later, I received my M.P.H. in epidemiology. My thesis was on pancreatic cancer in the Beaumont/Port Arthur area of Texas, and, to this day, the data have not been published. They lie on my shelf in a neat but faded green binder. This sobering, mentorless experience has driven me to encourage all my undergraduate and graduate students to select realistic topics for their theses/dissertations and to consider the work as just a beginning rather than as a career in itself. I always tell them, "You need to finish off, grow up and get on with the rest of your life."

Next I needed a job. I interviewed for a position as an occupational physician for Texaco, Inc., and was flown to their headquarters in White Plains, New York. They offered me the job, with a handsome salary and benefits, but were inflexible about my hours. In another snap decision, I rejected the offer. Instead, in 1981 I took a position at M. D. Anderson as an assistant professor, non-tenure track, part time, under Dr. Guy Newell in the newly created Department of Cancer Prevention and Control, which was then within the Division of Medicine. Guy Newell hired me purely on faith. My resume was one page, double-spaced. Besides Guy, there was only one other faculty member in the department. There was no infrastructure at all. My office was a cubicle in the former kitchen facility for the Texas Medical Center (now the Smith Research Building).

Shortly after I arrived in my new department, we received a phone call from a patient with salivary gland cancer who reported that a co-worker in his factory also had been diagnosed with the same malignancy; he wondered whether there was a common causative occupational exposure. Of course, I had no sage answer for him, but this gave me an idea. Over the next year, I and two unpaid but supremely dedicated research volunteers reviewed and abstracted the medical records of 329 patients with salivary gland cancer and a similar number of matched controls with other diagnoses. As we were analyzing these case-control data, a new chief of Pathology arrived at M. D. Anderson: Dr. John Batsakis, a world authority on the pathology of salivary gland cancer. I was in the right place at the right time. But, as I tell my junior faculty, you also have to *recognize* that you are in the right place at the right time. Otherwise, it turns out to be neither.

Together, Dr. Batsakis and I wrote and had three manuscripts accepted in the early 1980s, and, thus, my career as a cancer epidemiologist was launched. Many years later, I had the opportunity to send reprints of these three papers to Dr. du Plessis, the former professor of surgery whose internship I had so arbitrarily spurned years before. Surgical treatment of these tumors was his specialty. We exchanged some very meaningful letters that I have treasured. All was forgiven!

When Dr. T. C. Hsu, a brilliant cytogeneticist, approached me soon afterwards to help validate a new assay, the mutagen sensitivity assay he had developed to assess cancer susceptibility, I jumped at the opportunity. However, at that time I knew nothing about grant applications. No one had ever suggested I write and submit one. Moreover, I had no idea what a study section was, either. Could it be a chapter in a book? I did not understand anything about the workings of the National Cancer Institute (NCI) or the peer review process. Fast forward to the present — I have just completed two years on contract to the NCI, spending 10 percent of my time there working with both intramural and extramural scientists, and I'm now thoroughly conversant with the system. But I did prepare a small grant (my first) with Dr. Hsu to evaluate his assay in patients with head and neck cancer, and, with beginner's luck, it was funded. This turned out to be one of the earliest molecular epidemiology studies. We did not even recognize then that we were at the head of the curve.

I was so excited by this heady feeling of success that I jumped into the fray again and quickly submitted another grant. This time, it did not receive a fundable score. I was devastated, stuffed the review in the back of a drawer and never resubmitted that grant! Now, I insist that all faculty develop thick skins and that every grant, even those unscored, needs to be revised and resubmitted. And since I had no help in revising, I make it my top priority to participate actively in all the grant revisions in my department.

Next, there was an announcement from the NCI for grants on minority populations. By then, Guy Newell and I had published data showing that, in 1984, lung cancer overtook breast cancer as the leading cause of cancer mortality in Texas. Much the same trend was being shown in other states. We also documented that African-Americans had higher rates of lung cancer and earlier ages of onset (despite lower smoking intensity) than their white counterparts had. Exploring the reasons for these trends in minority poulations seemed to be a winning approach and, as a result, our lung cancer program was created.

I felt very insecure about this lung cancer grant application, my first R01. Several other applications on this topic were also being submitted from M. D. Anderson. I needed a new twist. I happened to go to Employee Health for a TB test, and sitting next to me, also waiting his turn, was Dr. Jack Roth, chairman of the Thoracic Surgery department. We discussed some ideas and devised a plan to look at germline changes in the tumor suppressor gene p53 as a risk factor for lung cancer. A few months later, my NCI program officer called to tell me that my grant was approved for funding. (There was no electronic communication in those days.) I was so amazed that I assumed Reagan's doctrine of "trust but verify" and called him back to verify that he had not made a mistake. How naïve I was then.

The lung cancer grant has been continuously funded now for 17 years. We showed that as many lung cancers were occurring in former smokers as in current smokers, and this gave my great friend and supporter, Dr. Waun Ki Hong, the brilliant idea to launch an innovative chemoprevention program in former smokers.

One sour note. A leading oncologist opined publicly that epidemiologic research, and mine in particular, was "phenomenologic." I had not heard the word before, and there was no Google engine then to search for the meaning. Could he have meant "phenomenal"? I did not think so, since I had detected a sarcastic undertone. I have spent the years since then striving — I believe successfully — to prove him wrong.

I have been extraordinarily fortunate in my career. As I walk through the expansive and bustling fourth floor of the Cancer Prevention Building, I not infrequently experience a flood of incredulity. Is this really the "house that I, as the founding department chair, helped build from its foundation?" I am exceptionally proud of the achievements of my department and its national reputation. I am equally proud of the talented and hard-working faculty, whose success is my success. I feel gratified that epidemiology is no longer considered a peripheral discipline but is now integral to most ongoing SPORE programs and many multidiscplinary programs throughout the institution.

I have been the recipient of many honors and awards, both at M. D. Anderson and nationally. Among the most meaningful are the Award for Research Excellence in Epidemiology or Prevention, from the American Association of Cancer Research and the American Cancer Society, and the Rosalind Franklin Award for Women Scientists, from the NCI. That this honor came from Dr. Joseph Fraumeni, whom I have so admired and whose textbook on Cancer Epidemiology became my bible early in my career, made it even more special.

I have learned everything I know on the job. I have met many amazing oncologists, surgeons, scientists, and of course, epidemiologists. I have learned so much from them: the importance of networking; how to prepare and edit a manuscript; how to make a formal presentation; to strike just the right tone in responding to a reviewer's critique; to be a gentle but decisive mentor; and to be honest but fair. I had to learn how to juggle and prioritize my life as a mother and wife with the realities of an academic career. I am, therefore, exquisitely sensitive to the special challenges facing our women faculty. I have made many mistakes but hope that I have learned from all of them to do better next time. I have never placed my own career needs above the needs of my children. That my daughter is now "having it all" as a devoted mother and extremely successful practicing radiologist is my ultimate success story.

Most recently, I decided, after much soul searching, to submit my name as a candidate for the position of head of the Division of Cancer

Prevention and Population Sciences to replace Dr. Bernard Levin, who was retiring. Then, I had second thoughts. It was not the right time for me personally. It was not the right time for my department to undergo a transition in leadership. Would the extensive changes I wanted to implement be acceptable to all? I was ambivalent. But I received an unexpected call from Dr. Margaret Kripke, then the Executive Vice President for Academic Affairs, informing me that I was one of the three candidates on the short list. My instincts jumped into high gear, and I told her that I was withdrawing my name. Once again, until I said it, I did not realize that I had already made this decision. I feel good about this decision, but time will tell all.

Postscript: In reviewing what I have written, I may have left you with the impression that my whole life has been nothing more than a series of impulsive decisions. This is not so. As I have gained wisdom and perspective, I have come to the realization that these life-changing moments were, in fact, *not* spontaneously arrived at. Rather, they were deliberate decisions reached in the deepest recesses of my mind, only waiting to be expressed. I am, after all these years, still a pragmatist.

Louise Connally Strong, M.D.

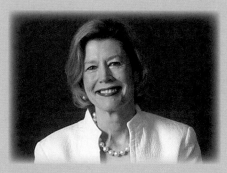

Professor of Genetics
Sue and Radcliffe Killam Chair

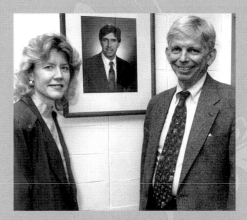

Louise has fond memories of mentor
Al Knudson, M.D., Ph.D.,
who accepted her for a postdoctoral
fellowship at M.D. Anderson in the
early 1970s.

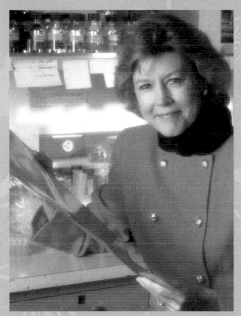

Collaborating with colleagues in their
laboratories helped Louise conduct
landmark studies to detect faulty genes
that predispose members of certain
families to cancer.

(Photo by Beryl Striewski)

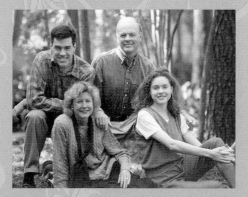

Posing for a family photo was fun
for Louise and husband Beeman
Ewell Strong III, their son Beeman
and daughter Larkin.

grew up in Houston in the 1950s, in a traditional home in which my mother was a primary homemaker (chief cook and bottle washer, chauffeur, seamstress and volunteer) and my father was not only the breadwinner but also my first and primary mentor. My older brother and I were always encouraged to excel in whatever we did and to believe that with hard work we could accomplish anything we set out to do. Our parents were big advocates of education, and I knew that I would have their support to pursue whatever path I chose. (They may have had second thoughts when I decided to apply to medical school!) We lived in the area now known as the Memorial Villages — before there were villages with city water and sewerage — and had horses, ducks, chickens, dogs and other animals. For years, my horse was my best friend, and I spent many hours riding throughout the undeveloped areas that now are filled with homes and many cars. My family has deep roots in Texas going back at least four to five generations. My father's family was primarily made up of lawyers, including my father, who served as a Federal District Judge from 1949 until his death in 1975; his father had represented Texas in the U.S. Congress, initially in the House and then in the Senate, from 1928 until 1956. My mother's family was primarily in medicine. Although I never knew my maternal grandfather, I heard many stories about his being the first pediatrician in Texas (he was allergic to the rubber gloves used in surgery so he "failed" in the family tradition of surgery and instead entered the emerging field of pediatrics).

I enjoyed high school, had excellent teachers, studied hard, and was a National Merit Scholar and a valedictorian of my graduating class at Lamar High School. I liked and was good at math, something of a social problem in the days when it was always announced before handing out scores that boys were expected to do well in math, and girls, in verbal skills. I always hid my reverse scores. And although I considered several colleges, I chose to follow in my father's and brother's footsteps at The University of Texas. The timing was great — as an avid football fan, I was there when the UT Longhorns played in their first national championship in 1963.

Though I majored in mathematics, I found myself increasingly interested in biology and genetics, both outstanding programs at UT. I knew I didn't want to be another lawyer in the family! I considered a Ph.D. in genetics, but none of the programs focused on human genetics, so I opted for medical school and enrolled in The University of Texas Medical Branch at Galveston (UTMB) in 1966 with the long-term goal of conducting research in human genetics. My first experience at M. D. Anderson Cancer Center came during the summer of 1967, when I received the Benjamin Stinnett Fellowship in Research Clinical Pathology and learned cytogenetics (human and other) with scientific giants T. C. Hsu, Ph.D., and Jose M. Trujillo, M.D., who became lifelong mentors, colleagues and friends.

Medical school for a woman in the 1960s in Galveston, an island off the upper Texas Gulf Coast, was pretty isolating. Women comprised about 5 percent of my class. Socializing and eating at the fraternity houses were not viable options. A friend and I made a pact to keep our sanity — we would play tennis every day no matter what! It might just be 30 minutes, but we would do it. And we did. Being on the island and working hard in a restricted setting, I somehow missed much of the turmoil of the 1960s. There were no marches and no protest movements in the medical school halls. However, I did manage to commute to Houston often enough to meet my future husband, Beeman Ewell Strong III, a UT undergraduate who had received his M.B.A. from Stanford University. He was working in Houston in the petrochemical business when he wasn't writing music or playing the guitar. (I remember how he embarrassed me by paging me throughout the John Sealy Hospital for a date.) We married in January 1970 before my graduation from UTMB that June and spent the first six months living on nearby Jamaica Beach. It became a popular spot for Houston friends to spend the weekend. I still recall leaving home early Sunday mornings when I had to be at the medical school and carefully stepping over bodies sleeping on our floor, some of whom I never saw again. Beeman proudly supported me and was one of only two male spouses recognized at graduation. The next day, my father-in-law told me how proud he was of me for finishing medical school and then advised me that, now that it was done, I could get busy with the important business of taking care of my family.

Since my first experience at M. D. Anderson, I had been thinking about cancer. While taking an elective in pediatric oncology there in 1968, I became interested in the etiology of childhood cancer — how could a child have cancer? Ultimately, this question led to my notion of joining two separate interests, genetics and childhood cancer, into a research program. As few thought genetics had anything to do with cancer in the 1960s, it could have been a tough sell. In 1969, I sought advice from the Office of Education at M. D. Anderson and met the director, Alfred G. Knudson, Jr., M.D., Ph.D., who also was dean of The University of Texas Graduate School of Biomedical Sciences (GSBS). I had no idea what he worked on, but I asked him about the possibility of developing a research program in genetics and childhood cancer. He smiled and said he was also interested in that topic and that perhaps I could do a postdoctoral fellowship with him. I have often wondered where I would have gone had he not been in his office that day!

Upon receiving my medical degree, I spent two years in a fellowship with Al Knudson. He had completed his now-landmark two-hit mutation model for retinoblastoma, based on age at tumor onset in heredity and non-heredity retinoblastoma. My project was to determine whether the two-hit model fit other childhood tumors. We worked first on Wilms' tumor of the kidney. It was very exciting when, in that pre-computer analysis era, together we plotted *by hand* the semi-log graphs of the ages at diagnosis for each Wilms' tumor patient group. We found a pattern similar to that of retinoblastoma. Al and I submitted the manuscript for publication in 1971, and Al departed for Europe for a month. Since that was before electronic communications and faxes, he told me that if the reviews came in during his absence, I should make revisions. Soon after he left, three reviews were returned. There was a short positive review, a short very negative review, and one with detailed suggestions that the research needed more work. Al's assistant indicated she had never seen such a negative review of his work before. I agonized about what to do and rewrote almost every sentence using "suggestive of" rather than our originally confident "demonstrated that" statements. Somewhat to my amazement the manuscript was accepted and published! My first!!

I continued working with Al on neuroblastoma and other childhood cancers until, just as my fellowship ended, there was a brand new focus in my life. I was pregnant! My son, Beeman Connally Strong, was born in May 1973, and I took a rather extended maternity leave. Motherhood was very compelling, and my career goals became cloudy. However, one day Al called to tell me of some exciting new reports. With the advent of chromosome banding and identification of individual chromosomes, Janet D. Rowley, M.D., had reported that the G group chromosome involved in Downs Syndrome (#21) was not the same as the G group chromosome involved in chronic myelogenous leukemia (#22, the Philadelphia chromosome), and, further, that the Philadelphia chromosome was not just a deletion but a translocation. I decided that I wanted to be part of the future of cancer genetics and came back to work part time for the next two years, which carried me through my second pregnancy and the birth of our daughter, Larkin Louise Strong, in November 1974.

Working full time with two small children was harder than I ever anticipated. I was excited to be back in research and foolishly accepted every speaking or writing opportunity that came my way, only to find that I could not handle all the commitments. I experienced a period of recurrent pneumonias over the period of 1976-1978, but eventually I was able to reorder my priorities, have more help at home, and accept that I could not "do it all." (With my X-rays in hand, I finally was able to demonstrate that I was at high risk and should get the pneumococcal vaccine and flu shot generally reserved at that time for the elderly or immune suppressed.)

On returning to work in 1975, I was invited to a National Cancer Institute (NCI) meeting on Genetics of Human Cancer. Having been relatively inactive for several years, I was thrilled to participate and meet others in the field. After giving my talk under very trying circumstances (my father had just died), I was invited to speak at the National Cancer Advisory Board in 1976. That opportunity was fortuitous because at the meeting a new NCI committee was proposed: the Clearinghouse for Environmental Carcinogens. I was asked to serve on the Data Evaluation/ Human Risk Assessment Subcommittee and did so from 1976-1980. That was the beginning of a long history of almost continuous NCI service.

Also, in 1975, I began to develop an independent research program, initiating a series of studies that continue to this day. In addition to Al Knudson, others who have been significant mentors include David E. Anderson, Ph.D., who shared his office space and resources with me until his retirement in the 1990s, and NCI investigators Robert W. Miller, M.D., Joseph F. Fraumeni, Jr., M.D., and Frederick P. Li, M.D. The NCI epidemiology program on childhood cancer etiology from the 1960s on provided many insights and ideas that have inspired me. I had some funding from a National Institutes of Health (NIH) Medical Genetics Center grant that I used to continue research on retinoblastoma and Wilms' tumor and, following on the work of Li and Fraumeni (1969), initiated a study of cancer in the families of children with soft tissue sarcoma. Li and Fraumeni had demonstrated that there were rare families with unusual patterns of early-onset and multiple primary cancers, distinctly unlike most recognized hereditary cancer syndromes at the time (now referred to as Li-Fraumeni syndrome or LFS). Although the etiology of this syndrome was unknown, I felt that we could further characterize it by studying families of M. D. Anderson patients, hypothesizing, of course, that it was genetic. In this pre-computer and pre-HIPAA (Health Insurance Portability and Accountability Act) age of 1975, we set out to locate the families of childhood sarcoma patients treated at M. D. Anderson from 1944 to 1975. Amazingly, we were able not only to locate the families but also to recruit them to our studies, to document reported cancers, and to develop extended pedigrees. These families have been spectacularly supportive of the research.

In the 1980s, my children were growing up, and life was busy with all the family activities. There were frequent conflicts — we didn't have synchronized electronic personal and professional calendars, so there were occasional missed events with family or late cancellations to meetings. Why were there always NCI advisory board meetings in Bethesda on the Monday after Mother's Day? I also endured the comments by my children that I was not a "normal" mom or an outburst by my daughter that she "would not want my life." But, overall, it was a positive time both personally and professionally.

We were successfully funded to continue our childhood cancer studies. I was awarded tenure and promoted to associate professor and, later, to professor. In addition, there were unexpected awards, some possibly a rare benefit of being female in a male-dominated faculty. In 1981, I received a letter from Charles A. LeMaistre, M.D., then president of M. D. Anderson, that I had been appointed to the Sue and Radcliffe Killam Professorship; I was the first woman faculty to receive an endowed position. It was a big surprise and honor, since I didn't know such positions existed. A few years later, the professorship was upgraded to the Sue and Radcliffe Killam Chair, which I continue to hold. The Killams not only are generous donors, but they also have been special family friends. Then, in 1984, I received a message that the White House had called. *The White House?* When I called back, I was told by a very impatient voice that President Reagan wanted to appoint me to a six-year term on the National Cancer Advisory Board. I had a few days to consider the offer. Everyone I asked said "take it," so as a young associate professor I did. The other woman scientist on the NCAB was Gertrude (Trudy) Elion, who in 1988 won the Nobel Prize in Physiology or Medicine. Serving on the NCAB was the beginning of six years that introduced me to some wonderful people and to the finances and policies of the NCI. Later in 1984, I received the Texas Federation of Business and Professional Women's Award for Outstanding Achievement in the Field of Oncology. As a multi-generation Texan, I was intrigued to learn that BPW members had a huge role in getting M. D. Anderson established by the Texas Legislature in 1941. Over the years, the BPW has actively supported cancer research conceived and conducted by our women faculty.

My research continued to focus on childhood cancer genetics, primarily retinoblastoma, Wilms' tumor and Li-Fraumeni syndrome, with longitudinal follow-up of families and application of new evolving technology brought by many creative collaborators to unravel the genetics. In addition, as childhood cancer treatment changed and became more successful, I participated in collaborative studies of long-term survivors of childhood cancer, a growing body of individuals who have significant late effects from the treatment. We have been able to maintain continuous NIH funding for these studies in various forms, most notably a P01 (program project grant) from 1984 to the present. Long-time M. D. Anderson collaborators have included the late Grady F. Saunders, Ph.D., for mapping of the Wilms' tumor and aniridia genes; Michael J. Siciliano, Ph.D., on studies of mutation and genome instability; Vicki D. Huff, Ph.D., on studying familial Wilms' tumor and mouse models; Guillermina (Gigi) Lozano, Ph.D., on p53 in human and mouse models; Christopher I. Amos, Ph.D., on statistical genetic analysis, and Michael A. Tainsky, Ph.D. (now at the Barbara Ann Karmanos Cancer Institute), for immortalization and tumorigenesis. Outside collaborators, especially in statistical analysis, include the late Wick Williams, Ph.D., and Ed Lustbader, Ph.D., both from Fox Chase Cancer Center. I also am grateful for the special relationship with the Retina Research Foundation, a Houston organization founded by Alice R. McPherson, M.D., from whom I have had funding to study retinoblastoma since 1982.

My research highlight to date was the finding of germline mutations in the tumor suppressor gene TP53 underlying LFS. During the 1980s, it had become clear from clinical and statistical data that these rare families seemed to have an inherited cancer susceptibility likely due to a single gene. The question was which gene. Several observations combined to make p53 a strong candidate. Michael Tainsky and I collaborated with Li and Fraumeni and with the laboratory of Stephen H. Friend, M.D., Ph.D., to identify mutations in p53 in the first five of five families studied. This was an important and highly visible scientific finding, published in the journal *Science* in 1990. But that is not why it is my "highlight." It was an overwhelming, almost scary feeling to know "the gene" for which a minor change could produce such a devastating effect and to realize that I knew such vital information about our research participants that they did not know about themselves. Almost immediately, the NCI held a conference to bring together ethicists, clinicians of many types (screening, diagnosis, treatment, prevention), geneticists, behavioral scientists, lawyers and genetic counselors to examine how we could effectively use this powerful new information. One of our research participants attended as a patient advocate. Issues of testing children, of imaging, of legal implications and other concerns were discussed, and guidelines for testing and counseling developed. At M. D. Anderson, we developed a research program to provide educational materials, counseling and testing to our research participants, and to determine what information people at risk wanted and how it would be used. The initial uptake on testing in the 1990s was low, although it has increased significantly since 2000. A personal benefit, and highlight, of this effort has been the opportunity to reconnect with the families who have been participants (in fact, almost collaborators) over the years. Many I knew from the 1970s, others I knew only from the telephone and the pedigrees. For some, I know the history for four to five generations. I've been privileged to share their histories and to see their families grow over another generation. These wonderful people have been my professional family. And now, finally, we had information that we could give back. We were able to bring family members together to discuss the risks with a genetic counselor and in some cases to take preventive measures. Unfortunately, given the range of tumors that occur with LFS, we have not been able to offer effective screening recommendations. For some, the genetic information is unwanted or seems more a burden than a benefit. The biggest disappointment to date is that we still do not have proven effective preventive/surveillance/management strategies for the individuals at risk.

For me personally, the 1990s brought the "empty nest," as my children went off to college. It had been fun to visit several schools with them, see the campuses, and, more important, see how they made decisions about continuing their education. My son went to UT, majoring in electrical engineering and computer science, and my daughter to Middlebury College, then Brown University, majoring in biology. Somehow college brought a blissful end to the teenage period and restored the closeness and communication of earlier years.

I had some interesting opportunities arise in the 1990s. M. D. Anderson had initiated a program of Faculty Achievement Awards, and I received the first award in Cancer Prevention. I became involved in the new Faculty Senate, the faculty governance body mandated by the UT System. This experience was very valuable; we (faculty) often see the institution through the tunnel vision of our day-to-day activities and associations, unaware of the many other faculty and missions that go on in other sectors. The Faculty Senate is the one organization that brings together an elected body from all departments and divisions and addresses faculty issues from the "faculty as a whole" perspective. While there have been many notable accomplishments of the Faculty Senate, clearly one from which I and probably others in this book benefit is the compensation review that initially revealed a pattern of strikingly lower salaries among women and minorities.

Outside the institution, there were also new opportunities. Like many other faculty at M. D. Anderson, I was a member of the American Association for Cancer Research (AACR), which is the largest cancer research organization in the world. It is the one professional organization that brings together all disciplines in the broad cancer research community with a focus on communication and fostering of science and public education. After being elected to the AACR Board of Directors, I became president in 1996-1997. One of the goals of my year was public education about cancer — not the media or marketing hype, but the current status and potential. At the annual meeting, we held the first public education session to provide a forum of experts to exchange information with the public, to present the opportunities and to hear the public concerns. This was a pilot; we had no idea what the level of interest might be on a Saturday morning, and didn't know whether to expect a handful or hundreds of participants. Fortunately, our local organizers in San Diego did a great job and really brought out the public. We had a full house with attendees staying beyond the scheduled time and thanking us for the session. It was terrific, people were so interested and so grateful, and we were touched. Those sessions now are standard at AACR annual meetings.

Of course, education is always an important part of academics. Over the years, I have been on many graduate students' committees. Often I have partnered with my laboratory collaborators, recommending that the students seek mentors with a "wet lab" so they can learn marketable skills but work with projects on which I am a collaborator. This approach was especially productive with the Grady Saunders lab. Students and postdocs who have contributed significantly to my program directly include Melissa L. Bondy, Ph.D., Sara S. Strom, Ph.D., Li Cheng, Ph.D., and Shih-Jen Hwang, Ph.D. I find that teaching is such an essential part of academic life; so many times in preparing a lecture or answering a student's question, I come up with a new idea or new hypothesis to test.

During the 1990s, new cancer genes involving relatively common cancers were identified, beginning with the breast cancer susceptibility genes BRCA1 and 2. These findings initially drove the development of clinical cancer genetics, a service offering genetic counseling and testing to concerned individuals. Over the last two decades, many new cancer susceptibility genes have been identified and rapidly incorporated into the program, and many students have trained in cancer genetics counseling. I very much enjoy working with the counselors but have to remember that my "historic approach" may not be so fascinating to everyone. The new trainees can't remember a time when we didn't know about such genes!

My most rewarding personal experiences have been from my family: with my husband, seeing our son and daughter grow up, graduate from college, get married, enter promising careers, start their own families — and, most important, maintain a close relationship with us. Our children are great individuals, and we have learned so much from them. This past year has brought the thrill of grandparenthood. On graduating from UT, my son took a job in Portland, Oregon, with Intel in chip architecture and design. Initially, we thought that would last a few years, and that he would, of course, come back to Texas. However, he has become an Oregonian, and we have loved getting to know Oregon. We anticipate increased visits there since he and his wife, Kirsten Healey, an artist and teacher, in April 2008 welcomed our second grandchild, a precious little boy named Beeman Driscoll Strong.

At one time it appeared that we would not have any Strong descendents in Texas. My daughter Larkin had moved from the northeast (Providence, Rhode Island) to the northwest (University of Washington in Seattle) in 2001 for graduate school. While there she met her husband Paul Scheet, also a graduate student, who was studying statistical genetics. They completed their Ph.D.s in health services/public health (Larkin) and statistics (Paul) in 2006 and moved to Ann Arbor, Michigan, for postdoctoral fellowships. In December 2007, they had our first grandchild, a beautiful little girl named Linnea Connally Scheet. I have to admit that I never knew I would be so excited about being a grandmother, but it is absolutely thrilling. I spent most of December in Michigan — and I really don't like cold weather — and returned to babysit in February. The great news for me is that Paul and Larkin completed their postdocs and joined M. D. Anderson in the summer of 2008 in the Department of Epidemiology. Imagine the joy of coming to work in the morning with the possibility of running into your daughter or son-in-law when the elevator opens or in the lunch line. And imagine stopping off on the way home to play with your granddaughter!

My career has not followed the traditional academic mode. I broke a cardinal rule: instead of the usual movement from one institution to another in an effort to advance up the career ladder, I have been at M. D. Anderson my entire career, without even a sabbatical. Perhaps had I been better informed about the "traditional" career path and what one needed to do to succeed, I would have considered other opportunities. And yet I have been happy with my research, and my choice worked for me and my family to stay in Houston. It certainly worked for my science, as I could never have conducted the longitudinal studies of M. D. Anderson patients and families elsewhere. It also worked as new technologies were developed and applied rapidly over these years at M. D. Anderson. I have had the fantastic opportunity to do what I loved without worrying about the "establishment" career path. One could hardly ask for more.

Peggy T. Tinkey, D.V.M.

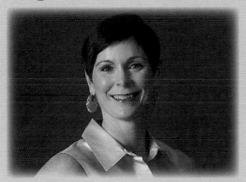

**Associate Professor and Chair
of Veterinary Medicine and Surgery**

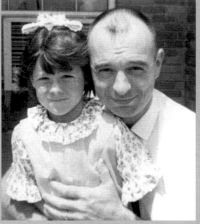

At age 5, Peggy probably was thinking about following in the footsteps of her veterinarian father Gale Taylor, D.V.M.

Peggy volunteered as a Candy Striper while in high school in San Antonio.

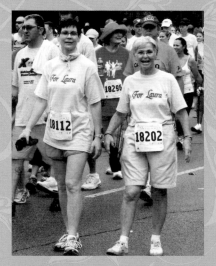

Mom Marilyn Taylor, right, joined Peggy for the 2007 Komen Race for the Cure; they walked in memory of Laura Britz, a family friend who had died from breast cancer.

y choice of career as a veterinarian was no real surprise to me or to anyone in my family. I guess you could say I was born into this profession because my father is a veterinarian. Added to that now are my brother and I, who both chose to follow in my father's footsteps and pursue a career in veterinary medicine.

As a child, I was surrounded by veterinarians — my dad, his colleagues and friends. I was steeped in a climate in which my professional role models were veterinarians, and I liked the vibe. Now (as then), the general public holds veterinarians in high regard and seems to view them with a certain mystique — we are "the gentle doctors." Maybe it's because our patients can't communicate verbally; maybe it's because they trust us implicitly and rely on us unfailingly to make the right decisions for them. I think all these things play a role in why the profession of veterinary medicine is seen as an honorable pursuit.

The odd bent in my career was my choice of a specialty in laboratory animal medicine. Since this is also my dad's specialty, you would expect that fact to have significantly influenced my decision, but it really didn't. His influence extended primarily to my selection of the profession itself. When a member of the general public conjures up an image of a veterinarian, they see the traditional practitioner, working in an office or on a farm, treating companion animals or livestock. Most people don't envision a laboratory scientist wearing a white lab coat and having rats and mice as the principal patients. It's this aspect of my career that most people find both fascinating and puzzling. The question that often springs from their lips is: "Why would you want to work on rats when you could be healing people's pets?"

Indeed, the choice of laboratory animal medicine as a career is not easily understood. As a laboratory animal veterinarian at M. D. Anderson Cancer Center, I provide veterinary care for animals used in cancer research here. My job comprises three major functions: providing an appropriate environment and clinical care for animals, ensuring regulatory compliance, and collaborating on research. Most of my professional colleagues are now Ph.D.s or M.D.s, and most of my patients are rodents. I work in a world where I am neither fish nor fowl — not a traditional basic science researcher and not a physician-clinician. Although my training is in veterinary medicine, most of my scientific contribution is in human medicine. It begs the question: Why would someone want to be the odd man out, the square peg in the round hole for most of his or her career? The answer is complex. For me, the simplest answer is that I fill a unique role that feeds my soul and suits my temperament. My skill set is unique and spans medicine, business management, regulatory compliance, research collaboration and mentoring. My love for animals is reflected in my dedicated commitment to their humane use in biomedical research. I act as the animals' advocate in a high-stakes world of animal research and medical progress.

The most important thing my parents did for me was to instill in me an appreciation for the value of education. My mom and dad were born in Illinois in the early 1930s and grew up in working-class families. They were not poor, but neither family was well off. Although none of my grandparents had a college education, they encouraged their children's education and supported their plans. My dad attended the University of Illinois and obtained his degree in veterinary medicine. During his years there, he met and married my mother. My mom was a good student in high school but had no plans to attend college. As a high school graduation gift, however, she received the money for one year's tuition at the University of Illinois from a favorite aunt and uncle. It was during that year that she met my dad. She never finished her degree because they got married and she quit school to work and support him while he finished school. When I received my bachelor's degree in 1981, I was the first person in my mom's family to graduate from college. I think my mom was prouder of that degree than I was — as soon as I received it, she took it and had it framed so I could proudly display it.

I decided in high school that I wanted to study medicine. Although I had not yet made a final decision about whether to pursue human or veterinary medicine, I decided to attend Texas A&M University because the only veterinary school in Texas was located there. I made the decision to apply to veterinary school during my freshman year at A&M. Mostly, this decision was based on my knowledge of the profession, since my dad is a veterinarian, and on my deep love of animals. Oddly, another thing that attracted me was the challenge. The competition for admission into veterinary school was and is fierce. I had been a high school athlete in track and basketball and loved the competitive challenge of athletics. I carried this competitive streak with me into the academic arena. The difficulty of gaining admission into veterinary school, rather than intimidating me, challenged and excited me.

My admission into Texas A&M coincided with a number of other firsts in my life. When I moved to College Station, it was the first time I had lived away from my parents' home; the first time I had to manage my finances, food, laundry and freedom; and the first time I had to live with roommates. I performed well academically, but I must admit that, for awhile, academic education took a back seat to all the other life lessons that I was learning. I was well prepared for university-level academics but less well prepared for the myriad of decisions that I was having to make about all other aspects of my life. I met a man, fell in love and got married — at the time, it seemed like the natural thing to do. I didn't struggle with the decision to get married or have children; these were things that I had wanted without question from

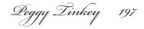

the time I was a child. In fact, I never remember even remotely considering the possibility that I might have to choose whether to forego children or marriage or family. That said, looking back it would have been better if I had used a bit more planning in the timing of those events. It is possible to have a marriage, family and career, but these things are big commitments and require focus, dedication, commitment, and lots of juggling of time and priorities for everyone for a long time. Thus, my decision to get married, have my son and start my first year of veterinary school at the age of 21, all within the same 12-month period, lacked insight. The biggest lesson that I learned during those years was that I gained an appreciation of the impact that the decisions of one spouse can have on a marriage. My decision to take on all those commitments affected my husband as well as me, and it was unfair and foolish of me to assume that he would feel the same way that I did about making the required sacrifices. As a result, we divorced while I was in veterinary school.

After learning from these experiences, my advice for young people is to focus on your long-term goals. I think it is especially important for women to realize that a successful marriage requires teamwork and that both partners must embrace those same goals. I know this is advice that young people have the least patience with and now find it amusing that this is exactly the advice that I chose to ignore during my early 20s. Although I wouldn't say that I regret my choices, I can see now that making different decisions would have made things much easier for me.

I pursued my veterinary education despite the turmoil in my personal life, and encountered several good mentors during veterinary school. A number of professors advised me on academic performance and career direction. During veterinary school, I worked part-time for Dr. E. Murl Bailey in the Veterinary Toxicology department and the laboratory animal research facility at Texas A&M. At that time, I was more interested in the paycheck than the career influence, but this early exposure to animal research had a significant influence later in my life. I learned about the use of animals in research and about the basic concepts of experimental methodology.

Dr. Claudia Barton, a veterinary oncologist in the small animal clinic at A&M, was another strong influence. I admired her professionalism and expertise, and she stimulated my early interest in cancer medicine. One of the things I admired most about Dr. Barton was her thorough knowledge of her subject. She seemed to know everything about any particular case in which she was involved. She knew the recent literature, the current theories and the recommended treatments, but more than that, she knew the owners' names, the pets' names and where they were from. Dr. Barton's professional life seemed to reflect the old saying, "If you're going to do something, then do it well." Slowly, through these experiences with my mentors, I was developing an appreciation and respect for professional and personal focus.

Amazingly, I never felt any gender discrimination while I was in veterinary school. My son was born mid-way through my first year of the program. During my last two years of veterinary school, I was a single mom, but I never felt that anyone treated me differently from any other student. However, it was also true that I didn't seek any special treatment; I only missed one week of school after the birth of my son, and I missed no more class time than any other students did. I made sure I was always prepared for classes and laboratories and was careful to pull my weight during night and evening clinic rotations. I had a couple of classmates who were loyal friends, and my parents provided tremendous moral and financial support.

Since completing school, my professional life has been divided between private veterinary practice and academic medicine. I spent 10 very rewarding years in private veterinary practice, and now have spent 14 years in academic medicine. Beginning my veterinary career in private practice seemed like the natural thing to do. Most people think of veterinarians as compassionately and carefully caring for people's pets, and I had that same mental image. I found practice very fulfilling. I loved interacting with pet owners and felt lucky to be able to enjoy many different animals. I have always loved animals, and this part of private practice fed my soul. Companion animals have so much personality; each of them is different, and I developed deep affection for many of my long-time patients.

I departed vet school fully armed with reams of theoretical knowledge and a modicum of practical knowledge about veterinary medicine. I knew anatomy, physiology, pathology, epidemiology — all the important "ologies" of animal medicine. I had developed skills — in animal handling, performing physical exams, auscultation, surgery — I thought I was ready!

And I *was* ready to interact with and treat my patients. But I soon discovered that I had a whole lot still to learn about how to interact with the humans who also were a part of my new career. I quickly discovered that most animal patients didn't walk through the front door of my practice by themselves (although some did, and that in itself is a good story). The vast majority of my patients presented as a human-animal duo, much like the chimera of Greek mythology. So I not only had to be concerned about the animals but also had to interact with and develop relationships with their owners, who came in all shapes and sizes. I also had to develop professional relationships with my boss, our employees, the boss's wife, the drug and equipment vendors, and my professional colleagues. I scanned my bookshelves and reviewed my class notes — where were the notes to help me with these things? How did I miss the class in interpersonal skills? Where was the textbook on business management, dealing with conflict, how to motivate employees, how to communicate in an emotionally charged situation? I quickly discovered that they don't call it "practice" for nothing.

Fortunately, I have a naturally agreeable personality and good innate interpersonal skills, and I found good support. I did not know enough to seek out specific leadership training while I was in practice, but I had good mentoring and advice from family and friends. We would discuss difficult situations that I encountered with clients, employees, friends, or family and I would soak in their advice. Also, after I left veterinary school, I remarried, this time to a fellow veterinarian who owned his own practice. Although he had no formal business training, he was a very good natural businessman, and I learned much from watching his style of management and discussing business decisions with him. I had been in private practice for 10 years when I changed directions in my career and entered the world of academic medicine as a laboratory animal veterinarian. By then, I had solid on-the-job training in client interaction, customer service and small business management. Life had prepared me, in quite an unplanned fashion, to take the next step in my career and personal development.

My initial step into an academic research institution was not dissimilar from private practice in many ways. I worked for a boss; provided health care for animals; supervised employees; and interacted with a variety of "clients" in the guise of research investigators, who "owned" the animals. The skills that I had learned in private practice served me well here, and I moved into positions of greater responsibility. In my new role, I benefited from another group of great mentors, who showed me the rules of the game required for success in an academic environment. In business, the end goal was always profit; whoever ran the most profitable business would be the most successful. In a state-owned, academic research institution, the rules for success are different. I learned that the rungs of my ladder were now promotion and/or tenure and that the criteria needed to qualify for advancement fell into three categories: service, teaching and scholarly contribution. Drs. Kenneth Gray and Cliff Stephens were colleagues in my department who served as wonderful mentors to me. "These three elements," my mentors explained, "make up the legs of a three-legged stool. You don't have to be equally strong in all three areas, but you must show achievement in all three to be successful." My skill set grew to include writing manuscripts, teaching students and staff, and mentoring junior colleagues. I loved these new challenges as much as I had loved the challenges of private practice, and I did well in this new environment. A major challenge was to achieve veterinary board certification in the specialty area of laboratory animal medicine, and I achieved this. I was promoted to associate professor and named deputy chairman of the department.

It was at this new level that I saw in sharper focus another distinct difference between a small business environment and academic medicine.

The chain of command in a small business is simple. There is a boss; there may be a few folks directly underneath the boss, and there are employees. The lines of reporting are very clear. This, however, is not the case in an academic environment. Although it is true that I reported to one boss on the organizational charts, that boss was also a peer of those who reported to him. Also, most decisions were preceded by a period of negotiation and review before they were finalized. Thus, the military style of leadership, which is often effective in small business, was not the most effective style in academic medicine. Effective leadership now required teamwork, building consensus, establishing group ownership and creating buy-in. These skills were not as easily learned through on-the-job training. M. D. Anderson's administration deserves much credit for recognizing this and implementing a faculty leadership program. My chairman recommended me for it, and that was the start of my first formal training in leadership skills.

I feel fortunate to have been treated fairly throughout the majority of my career. My sole experience with gender discrimination occurred when I interviewed for my first professional position. Soon after I accepted it, I learned that a male classmate had been offered the job first and had turned it down. He stated that the reason he was their top candidate was because he did not have personal commitments that might interfere with the job. I interpreted this to mean that although our academic and interpersonal skills were regarded as equal, I was considered the less desirable candidate because I was a single mom. While I understood the reasoning behind this, I still felt the innate unfairness of it. Although I have usually believed that I was judged on my ability, qualifications and experience rather than on the basis of my gender, the sting of that single experience gave me a glimpse of how unfair it is to be judged based on assumptions and personal prejudices.

In truth, the topic of how women can successfully balance the responsibilities between family and profession is a delicate matter and involves personal choice. For me, a professional education is a privilege, not a right. I believe that the recipient of such an education then has a responsibility to use it to help society. I also feel strongly that a person can have a professional career *and* a personal life and, moreover, that pressure to limit one's personal life due to work demands acts to the detriment of both the person and the workplace. I never felt that I had to choose between career and family; for me, these two aspects of my life complement each other. My career fulfills me and helps me grow as a person and, as a result, I'm a better parent. I think my children have benefited enormously from having parents with stimulating, interesting full-time careers that they love. My hope is that, as a result of this, my children have learned not to settle for a job that is "just for money" but rather to pursue their passions. I value the M. D. Anderson culture because the administration has made work-life balance a priority.

This reflects an environment that values whole people, and I choose to pursue my career in this type of caring, nurturing environment.

I have always thought it amusing that my ability to advance and achieve leadership roles seemed to owe more to my people skills than to my medical skills. Certainly, I am not discounting the value of my education — I realize that I would not have my position today if I were not a veterinarian with advanced training in laboratory animal medicine. However, my ability to simply get along well with others has always seemed to be one of the most appreciated traits in the workplace. I have found this ironic because, especially in the complex world of medicine and research, this ability seems so basic and simple. This is, in fact, not the case. Leadership is a learned skill, and the development of good leaders is absolutely essential for any organization to survive and thrive. M. D. Anderson has made a strong commitment to developing leaders among its faculty and staff. The Faculty Leadership Academy here had a huge impact on me because it gave me formal leadership training for the first time in my career. Although I had good natural interpersonal skills, I always felt uneasy with conflict and had become reluctant to pursue positions of authority because in those positions, managing conflict was inevitable. Instead of being an aggressive self-promoter who climbs the corporate ladder, I was "the reluctant leader." The leadership skills that I learned at the Faculty Leadership Academy gave me confidence to take on greater leadership roles. Also, I encountered other accomplished M. D. Anderson women whom I observed and admired: Drs. Margaret Kripke, Elizabeth Travis, Ellen Gritz, Margaret Spitz and Gigi Lozano. All of them served as role models; their success helped me gain the confidence I needed to take on the challenge of chairing a department.

I now feel that I'm entering the most fulfilling and productive years of my career and personal life. My son is married and in law school, and my daughter is a senior in high school and busy making plans for graduation and college. The research programs at M. D. Anderson have grown enormously over the past 10 years, and the challenge ahead is to maintain a world-class animal research program to support the institution's research efforts. I'm privileged to work with a faculty and staff of over 100 people who share this common goal. We're all committed to doing our part in "making cancer history." I bounce out of bed every morning and am excited about what the day will bring. It just doesn't get any better than this.

Elizabeth L. Travis, Ph.D.

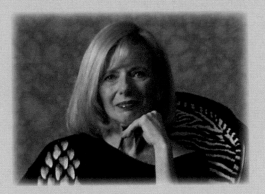

Associate Vice President for Women Faculty Programs
Professor of Experimental Radiation Oncology
Mattie Allen Fair Professor in Cancer Research

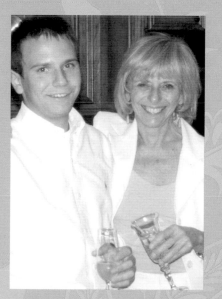

Elizabeth helped son Scott celebrate his graduation from Lamar High School in 2005.

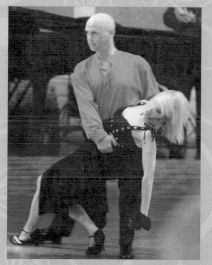

Elizabeth and her dance partner William were a big hit at the River Oaks Country Club, where they danced the tango at a Spotlight performance in December 2006.

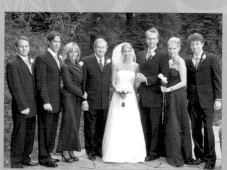

In October 2007, Elizabeth enjoyed the wedding of Jerry Hyde's daughter Sarah to John Williams. Flanking them at left were Elizabeth's son Scott and Jerry's son Jonathan, while siblings Anna and Stephen Hyde are at right.

(Scott Cramer Photography, Vail, Colorado)

s a young girl, I never imagined that I would one day be doing something that I love and get paid to do it. Growing up, my first loves were music and dance, and they still remain my passions, particularly dance. But as I went through school, I discovered that I also enjoyed studying and getting good grades. My father was an avid reader and I grew up in a home filled with books, so this love of learning was not too surprising. I was also highly competitive and a fierce spelling bee competitor in elementary school, a result of Sunday night Scrabble games with my family. Only straight A's were acceptable to my parents and me. The only class I managed to almost fail miserably was home economics — clearly an ominous sign for my domestic future!

I grew up in Wilmerding, Pennsylvania (population 5,000), one of those small, unremarkable mill towns 10 miles to the east of Pittsburgh. I am the older of only two daughters but was raised in a large Italian extended family with blurred boundaries between first and second cousins, aunts and uncles, and great aunts and uncles — we were all just family. I am a second-generation Italian-American (LaTorre is my maiden name) and proud of my heritage. I love being Italian! One of my goals is to speak the language fluently and spend at least three months a year in Italy when I retire.

My parents were born in this country, and both of them finished high school but neither went to college. My maternal grandfather built a small, successful family-run bar and grill in my hometown, and my maternal grandmother, a homemaker, also helped run the business. My father worked there full-time, and my mother, on weekends only. My father (now deceased) was a bartender (and a good one, since he was a good listener). My Mom always worked from home to supplement the family income. She was a seamstress with impeccable taste and made most of my sister's and my clothes. I credit her for my love of fashion! She did not work outside the home until I was 16. Although not a professional woman, she was the role model of a working mom for my sister and me. I had a happy childhood. Nevertheless, there were difficult times; money was not plentiful although my parents shielded us from their worries. They both were hard working (my mother, now 86, still works part time!), always striving to better the world of their family. Thus, my sister and I were taught a strong work ethic and to always "reach high."

I developed a love of problem solving in junior high school. One of my teachers during those years told my parents "Elizabeth should go to college!" Even though I was a straight-A student, my parents were a little surprised; they just had not thought about it. At that time, only three family members (my cousins) — all male — had graduated from college, although their sister had not. In fact, no *woman* in the family had attended college — I would be the first! But from then on, my parents' goal was that both of their daughters be college graduates (which we both are), although neither they nor I had any idea what that entailed besides a lot of money.

Though small, my hometown of Wilmerding prided itself on the excellence of its public schools. In high school, I chose the college track and in Mr. Smith's 10th grade biology class fell in love with science. He was an unforgettable teacher whose enthusiasm and love of science was so infectious that many of my classmates eventually chose medicine, science or engineering as a career — a testament to the power of one teacher to make a difference in the lives of young people.

So I wanted to study science and be a scientist, although I had no clue what that meant! But I remained drawn to the world of dance. I had taken dancing lessons from the age of 5 and, although I loved it, in the end I chose science. My goal was to attend the University of Pennsylvania, but my parents were more comfortable sending me to the same school that my three cousins had attended, Indiana State Teacher's College (now Indiana University of Pennsylvania) in Indiana, Pennsylvania. Of course, I was going to be a teacher because "You can always get a job if something happens to your husband!" I was excited about college and approached it with enthusiasm mixed with a little apprehension, but the excitement won!

I knew that I did not want to teach and dreamed of "working in a lab," but I nevertheless attended this college and took every science course available. And it was during these years that two remarkable things happened. First, my cell biology professor encouraged me to consider graduate school, which was back then a "black hole" to me. Second, I enrolled in an elective course in radiation physics and biology in my junior year — and I was hooked! Fate further intervened when, through my father's personal physician (who unbeknownst to us was a faculty member at the University of Pittsburgh Graduate School of Public Health in the Department of Radiation Health), I was offered a summer job in the lab he shared with his collaborator, Joe Watson. My dream of working in a lab was finally a reality.

So began the path that led to my current positions at M. D. Anderson Cancer Center, though the course was anything but linear. I meandered down a "long and winding road" in which fate and calculated risk-taking played major roles. After graduating from Indiana State College, I was accepted into the University of Pittsburgh Graduate School of Public Health, working in the lab of Joe Watson. However, before I could complete my master's degree, I married another graduate student (thus the name Travis) who became an officer in the Navy and was stationed in Charleston, South Carolina. Leaving Pittsburgh with him did not allow me sufficient time to complete my master's thesis in radiation biology, so I reluctantly settled for a master's in education rather than get no degree. At that time, long-distance marriages for professional reasons were unheard of. This was one of the few times in my life when I did what was expected of me. I realized that even if I were a teacher, my "primary" role would be wife and, probably, mother. I soon discovered that this was not the right road for me.

The first year I was in Charleston, I taught high school biology, just as my Dad had suggested, and found that I really enjoyed it. However, an opportunity to work in the Radiation Therapy department at the Medical University of South Carolina (MUSC) that summer took me down a different path. I just wanted to work in a lab again, but the department was looking for someone with a radiation biology background to set up a lab and design a course for the residents. I had no experience doing either of these things, but they offered me the job, and, despite my concerns that I was unqualified, I accepted. I assumed they were desperate, but I knew that I could only learn. Halfway through the summer, they offered me the position permanently, and I declined but immediately realized that I had forfeited a once-in a-lifetime opportunity. The next day, I sheepishly admitted to them that I would like to accept the position if it were still available. Taking this risk turned out to mark a pivotal point in my life and my career, and it is one of the major decisions that put me on the path to M. D. Anderson. The experiences, the opportunities, the people I met in the radiation oncology/biology world, the exposure to radiation as a treatment for cancer — all these were crucial to my career. During this time, I published my first major work, "Primer of Radiobiology," a textbook aimed at radiation technologists and radiology residents, for whom there was no appropriate text at that time.

To further sweeten the deal, I applied to the graduate school at MUSC for a Ph.D. in experimental pathology and studied with Rusty Harley, a pulmonary pathologist at MUSC. I considered returning to the University of Pittsburgh to study classical radiobiology with my former mentor, Joe Watson, but true to the meaning of the word "mentor," he sagely advised me that I would have more opportunities with a degree that married radiation biology with experimental pathology than I would have with a classical radiobiology degree, so I stayed at MUSC. The man had a crystal ball! Although the normal tissue complications of radiation therapy were well known, at that time there was increased interest in this area of radiobiology research, particularly for the so-called "late responding tissues," of which lung is one. The decision to pursue a Ph.D. in experimental pathology thus proved to be another pivotal career decision. Unfortunately, my marriage was a casualty of this period, so while pursuing my degree I continued to work, which prolonged the time to achieve my goal but allowed me to achieve it.

When I graduated from MUSC in 1976 with a Ph.D. in experimental pathology, I realized that this degree alone would not be sufficient to enable me to secure independent funding for my research and, further, that without more training in this field, I would never be taken seriously as a radiation biologist/pathologist. So, I applied for postdoctoral positions in world-class radiobiology labs. My Dad had always taught me that "they can say yes or no, but, if you don't ask, you won't get anything." I had begun to train my sights on M. D. Anderson for my future, as it was the home of Rodney Withers, an M.D. (pathologist) and Ph.D. and the leading expert in normal tissue radiobiology.

I wrote to a world-famous radiation pathologist at the Hammersmith Hospital who, unfortunately for me, was retiring at that time but graciously forwarded my letter to Jack Fowler, the director of the Gray Laboratory. Much to my amazement and surprise, Jack made me an offer, sight unseen, to come to the Gray Lab for one to three years in a position as a lecturer at the University of London, a fancy title for a postdoc. My training in pulmonary pathology was key, as the Gray Lab had begun to focus on radiation damage in less-studied normal tissues. I immediately accepted this opportunity to study in this world-renowned laboratory in my field — undoubtedly the single most important decision I made personally and professionally. The opportunity to live in England (I had never been abroad) and study at the Gray Lab was a dream come true! Again, I was absolutely certain that if I did not accept this opportunity, I would regret it and always wonder "what if?" I knew absolutely no one at the lab or in England for that matter, but that was unimportant. I have always had a sense of adventure.

Jack Fowler is a remarkable man, a terrific scientist, and an exceptional mentor and advocate. Jack taught me how to ask questions. Whenever I went to his office with an idea, he would say "What's the question?" He taught me about scientific inquiry, how to design experiments, and how to write papers. I learned finally what a scientist did and really how to do it. I was also surrounded by some of the best minds in the field at the time. My main goal was to become known as an expert in normal tissue radiation damage, specifically, radiation-induced pulmonary fibrosis and pneumonitis. With the help of many talented people in that lab, I succeeded in becoming known as Liz "lungs" Travis.

It was during this time that I encountered the first serious challenge in my career. While at the Gray lab, I developed a novel assay for radiation-induced lung damage that then represented a paradigm shift and was viewed with skepticism, if not outright disbelief. The paper was initially rejected, but I did further experiments and the work was subsequently published. The assay in question is now a standard technique in studying pulmonary injury after many types of insults. This experience taught me to persevere and to "do what is necessary to publish your data." To wit, the experiment is not finished until the data are out the door.

I stayed at the Gray Lab for all three years, living sometimes in rather awful conditions but knowing deep in my heart that this was the right thing to do. It was the experience of a lifetime and one that I will always cherish, both professionally and personally. I made friendships during this time that are sustained to this day. This was truly the training that positioned me for my recruitment to M. D. Anderson.

From the Gray Lab, I accepted a position in the Radiation Oncology department at the National Cancer Institute (NCI) in Bethesda, Maryland, and, then, in 1982 I was recruited to M. D. Anderson, another dream come true for me. M. D. Anderson had a long and outstanding reputation in normal tissue radiobiology, and I was honored to come here. I joined the faculty as an associate professor on the tenure track, was tenured in 1985, and was promoted to professor in 1988 — a career trajectory that I ascribe to my years at the Gray Lab and the NCI. I wrote grants, published papers, and had a wonderful lab with great technicians, students, postdocs and fellows. I really loved what I was doing and where I was doing it. Mostly, it was great fun. I was the only woman faculty member in the department.

Although married briefly, I had no desire to do so again, but I began to wonder whether I would be happy without children. I actually had never imagined myself as a wife and mother, but after my sister had a son, my psyche started churning, weighing the pros and cons of whether to have a child. My epiphany was actually driven by science and occurred the morning after a site visit for our P01 grant, the second one where I presented my research. The site visit went well, but it made me realize that science alone, as much as I loved it, would not be enough for me in life. So I decided to have a child and knew, yet again, deep in my heart and soul that if I did not do this, I would forever regret it. And I know this even more now that my son, Scott Phillips, is 21.

So how did I, a single mother and a professor with a busy lab, manage my household and career and raise a child? First, I made a clear decision that my son was a priority. Moreover, I decided that I was not going to miss out on this wonderful experience, especially as everyone told me how fast children grow up, and they were right. Convenience to the institution guided my lifestyle. We lived within two miles of the medical center in a family-oriented neighborhood complete with programmed summer activities for kids. Schools, doctors and dentists were all in proximity. The other necessities and tasks of daily life, such as housecleaning, yard work, etc., I paid others to do. Bottom line? Get as much help as you can afford. I started with a live-in nanny who also cooked dinner, a real lifesaver.

I also realized that I would have to prioritize my work life. For example, I carefully chose which out-of-town conferences to attend and which institutional committee appointments to accept. I tried to have breakfast and dinner with my son every day and considered early morning or late evening meetings to be decidedly family unfriendly. My office policy in my new position is "no meetings before 8 or after 5." I always tried to be home by 5 p.m., but the dinner hour got progressively later as Scott got older, and this is the only complaint he has ever vocalized about his working mom (though I am sure there are many more). As a survival tactic, he learned to cook and is a great cook, a highly desirable trait in a man! Because I am a night owl, I would work after he was in bed, but the hours between my arrival home and his bedtime were devoted to him. Still, he grew up with the impression that I worked too hard. I think one of my gifts to him is that he knows that I love what I do and that for me it was and is "not work." Scott is a rising senior at UT Austin in the McCombs Business School. He also loves what he is doing. My son is my legacy, and I would have been saddened to have missed the wonders of having and raising him. For me, it has been a thrilling, life-enhancing experience. Did I forfeit some career opportunities? Yes, but I always knew that I could not simultaneously grow a department and a child as a single mother. Knowing my priorities always made difficult decisions clearer, although not necessarily easier.

So I continued my journey here at M. D. Anderson, making this my scientific and professional home for my whole career. I have no regrets. During most of these years, my life was quite frankly centered on my son and my science, with the rest of my free time spent with friends and my family, with whom I am very close. My sister and her family and my mother live in Clearwater, Florida, and I still escape for a week each summer to visit them, sit in a cabana on the beach, eat grouper sandwiches, watch the water, and generally re-charge my batteries. I have discovered that there are certain things that are truly at your core; besides science, mine are lying on the beach, reading and dancing. I have learned to respect and to nurture this core.

When Scott left for college, I had time to resurrect my passion for dance, and I now take ballroom and Argentine tango lessons. Dancing feeds my heart and spirit and is also good for my body and a great stress reliever, although my competitive instinct and desire to do better rear their heads even in what is supposed to be just fun! I also was fortunate to meet a wonderful man, Jerry Hyde, who has nothing to do with science or medicine. We have merged our families — my son Scott and Jerry's four children! Now that all of the kids are out of the house, traveling is one of our favorite pastimes. Jerry has a wonderful sense of humor; at one event, he referred to himself as my "tenured" boyfriend, only to be reminded by my colleagues that our tenure is renewable!

At every phase of my career, I had mentors who were teachers, became friends and taught by example how to be a mentor. I have long appreciated and will always be grateful to those individuals, all male, who guided and taught me during this journey and had faith in me that I myself did not have, starting with my 10th grade biology teacher, my first mentor. My mentors at the Gray Lab taught me another valuable lesson: how to balance work and life and still maintain highly successful careers. They never forfeited vacation days! I am not sure why this seems to be impossible to do now.

Since my graduate education took place between 1970 and 1976, it is also not surprising that none of my mentors were women. All of my male mentors were wonderful, but the lack of female mentors who successfully combined science and a family did not provide a model for this lifestyle. Fortunately, this is not the case today, as many outstanding women physicians and scientists are able to blend a successful career with marriage and children, although it is still not easy. I "grew up" in science when gender bias was alive and well. My first real encounter with this issue was in graduate school at the University of Pittsburgh School of Public Health. In the program of 20 graduate students, I was one of only two women. Not all of the professors agreed that women belonged in science, and one in particular made it quite clear to both of us that he thought teaching us was a waste of his time and that we were taking up space that should belong to male students. This was an astonishing attitude, since the field of radiation sciences included Marie Curie, the only woman ever to receive two Nobel prizes.

I also encountered salary bias in one position, but my department chair rectified this after I questioned why he had offered a new male employee with the same credentials and experience as I had more money than I was making. His reason? "He (the male employee) has a family to support." Fortunately, such justification is no longer acceptable or legal. I was very uncomfortable having this "difficult conversation" with my chairman, especially because I was very junior, but its successful outcome has helped me conduct other difficult conversations that inevitably occur throughout a career. I encourage (and mentor) women faculty to have these conversations when necessary.

It was not until I went to the Gray Lab that I really worked with other women in science. Unfortunately, this, too, was not always a pleasant experience and actually surprised me. But women also have gender bias issues, a well-known phenomenon in our world. Even so, it was still refreshing to be around these wonderfully successful women, who were professional role models for me. Except at the Gray Lab, I was the only woman professional in the departments where I worked. This was the case both at the NCI and in my department at M. D. Anderson at the time of my recruitment. Today, my scientific department, Experimental Radiation Oncology, has 50 percent women faculty. I think that lone women in departments tend to isolate themselves from their colleagues for a variety of reasons. I did this to some extent because, as a single mother, I thought I did not have time for chatting, and I had to work fast and hard so I could leave by 5 o'clock with a minimum of guilt! That isolation proved to be a serious error in judgment and one that I urge busy women faculty not to repeat. When I needed supporters, there were none, and that was a painful experience.

My personal journey in science has in many ways been unconventional — full of twists and turns, good luck and calculated risk taking, coupled finally with determination about my goals and an awareness of how to obtain them. I am fortunate that my parents were always supportive throughout my wayward career, although occasionally skeptical of my choices. I have no pat answers for how to balance personal life and work or advice on the best time to have children. I had my child when I was a tenured professor, which allowed me more flexibility than as a graduate student, but having children past "prime time" in itself presents unique challenges and considerations. I can only suggest that you listen to your heart and your gut — in my experience, they have never let me down. Decide what's important and don't lose sight of it. But, mostly, love what you are doing.

Recently, I again followed my heart by accepting the position of Associate Vice President for Women Faculty Programs here at M. D. Anderson, a new endeavor that presents challenges different from those of running a research lab. My lab is still active and funded, but the scope of the work is reduced. My priority these days is to champion women faculty at the institution. I try to spend Fridays in the lab, as it remains my "roots," and I still derive pleasure and satisfaction from research. But I also feel that, for me, it is time to return a little of what this wonderful career has given me and to provide opportunities to help others achieve their full potential. I am fortunate and grateful for this new opportunity, in which my "day job" is once again something that I love doing and that I hope will make a difference in the lives of others.

Cheryl L. Walker, Ph.D.

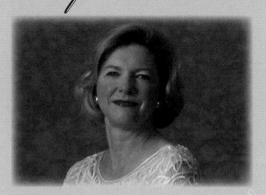

Professor of Carcinogenesis
Ruth and Walter Sterling Professorship

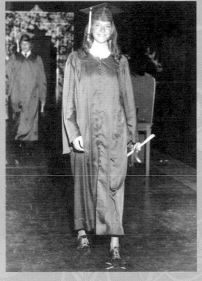

A happy Cheryl graduated from Sunset High School in 1973.

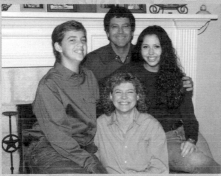

Cheryl and husband Mike sat with son Christopher and daughter Ashley for the family's 2001 Christmas card photo.

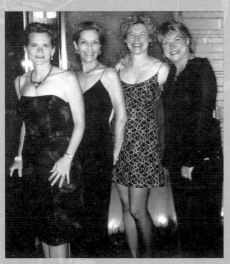

The 2005 "annual girls weekend" in New York City added another fun memory for this quartet, from left Cinda, Muriel, Cheryl and her sister Gail.

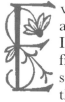ven if you didn't grow up in the South, if you are "of a certain age," you may in your youth have dreamed about your future, as I did in the wee hours of the many sleepovers with my girlhood friend, Becky Kilman. The dreams were of medical school and law school, not because these were to be our careers, but rather because these were the places where I would find my doctor husband and she her lawyer husband. The idea that we could actually have these careers ourselves never really entered our minds, but we were sure that these were perfect careers for our future husbands. Thankfully, the idea that if you are female, a career is strictly optional has now come and gone. But at that time and in our circumstances, this was how we were raised. I guess it is ironic that Becky actually did go on to law school at The University of Texas and that I went to UT Southwestern Medical School — and we both obtained our own professional degrees instead of finding lawyer or doctor husbands.

During the 1960s and 1970s, without careers to distract us, girls growing up in the South focused on being beautiful, popular and cheerleaders — or at least being on the drill team. As it turns out, as a young girl I was neither particularly adept at the necessary skills nor did I possess the physical attributes to easily be any of these. However, with lots of effort, by high school I did make the drill team, and although I certainly was not beautiful, my five closest friends grew up to be the five most beautiful girls in our high school. Thus, mostly by association, I came to be regarded as popular, too. On reflection, I now greatly value the people skills that I honed in striving for the adolescent acceptance that seemed so elusive at the time. I learned that being gracious, having a positive outlook, being enthusiastic (and smiling under stress, a drill team staple), and taking an interest in others attracted them to me. These attributes have continued to stand me in good stead as I interact with my colleagues today, and these skills (especially smiling under stress) have been invaluable as I have risen through the ranks to leadership positions in my profession.

As I grew up, my family's financial circumstances evolved from "modest" to "very well off" due to my father's success as an entrepreneur. When I was very young, he took a position as a department store buyer, an event that moved our family from Oregon to Dallas. He then went on to found two large and successful companies. We originally settled in the beautiful Oak Cliff neighborhood in Dallas; however, during the 1960s the area was undergoing a dramatic transition from a lovely enclave to a rundown and blighted neighborhood. As a result, by the time I reached high school our part of town comprised mostly disadvantaged families, with many teenagers from my neighborhood being bused to affluent schools in the northern parts of the city in order to achieve desegregation. "Dismal" is the best way to describe my high school education at one of the most underserved schools in the district. I'm sure I must have taken the college SAT, though sans any of the prep courses that I now know from my own children's experiences are obligatory and also without any appreciation of the importance of the test, which at the time just seemed like another annoying achievement test that required us to be at school on a Saturday. In fact, if my "underprivileged" high school had a college counselor, I never was aware of one. It was a real eye-opener when my own children attended high school, and I found that not only did high schools have college counselors but also their high school had three counselors for the senior class alone.

One exception to my otherwise inadequate high school education was a fantastic biology teacher named Mr. McKemie. I loved every aspect of his class, from the ubiquitous frog dissections to my first taste of Mendelian genetics. Growing up, I had never been a tomboy, but I *was* fascinated by nature. Like most kids in the 1960s, I played outside a lot, and the nearby woods and golf course creek were my constant haunts. Not only did Mr. McKemie ignite in me a love of biology that had been simmering below the surface, but he also was the only teacher that singled me out as a talented student. It was true that I was talented — I immediately grasped concepts that others found difficult — and Mr. McKemie even let me design experiments to work on after class. This time not only reinforced what I was learning in the classroom but also made me feel special in a way that I hadn't experienced before. It was this interaction with him and the realization and confidence that biology was something I was good at that led me to decide this should be my major in college.

As graduation approached, I was told by my parents, who were by then financially well off, that I could go to any college I wanted; however, this was only partially true. The reality was that I could go to any college that would accept me. Unfortunately, I had no clue about what constituted admissions criteria, and "Ivy League" was not even a part of my vocabulary. What I *did* know was that I had had a great time skiing on Young Life ski trips to Colorado with my church youth group, and since I remembered Denver as a beautiful mountain city in the snow, I thought Denver would be a great place to go to school. Thus, I applied to and was accepted at the University of Colorado. Imagine my shock when I arrived to start my freshman year at the university and found that the campus was in Boulder — *not* Denver!

While I was preparing for my first semester in college, an unanticipated benefit of my less-than-stellar high school education remarkably worked to my everlasting advantage. I had taken chemistry in high school, but this was a subject for which I had very little aptitude and one that was taught with little enthusiasm by Sunset High School's aging golf coach. Even *I* was aware that my knowledge of chemistry was not good enough for college if I hoped to get a degree in biology. Then, the summer after high school graduation, while lounging at the pool working on my tan (yes, I visit my dermatologist regularly!) and perusing the freshman course list, I noticed that there were two choices for freshman biology: "regular" biology (taught by professors from the Evolution, Population and Organismic Biology department) and "molecular" biology (taught by professors from the Molecular, Cellular and Developmental Biology department). I had never heard of molecular biology, but the course syllabus stated that in addition to molecular biology, "principles of chemistry will be covered." "Great," I thought, "a refresher course in chemistry!" So I blithely enrolled in freshman MCD biology, which turned out to be one of the hardest (and most wonderful) freshman courses offered at the university.

And, as it happened, in the 1970s the University of Colorado was one of the few universities in the country to have a department specializing in what was then the "emerging" field of molecular biology. The MCD biology department had stellar faculty, many of whom were in the National Academy of Sciences. As a freshman, I discovered that molecular biology was fascinating and that I had a natural affinity for it (despite having no knowledge of chemistry) — and *I was hooked!* To this day, I remember most of the professors and many of their lectures, and, although the molecular biology of the 1970s was rudimentary compared with today's science, at the time it was revolutionizing biology. Thus, the irony that participating in church ski trips and receiving a poor high school education ultimately landed me in one of the premier environments for learning molecular biology has not been lost on me. In truth, I consider it providential.

One of my great blessings is that I have been able to find success in a demanding career and still have the fulfillment of a close and loving family. I owe this entirely to my wonderful husband, who has been an equal contributor (and, truth be told, in many respects a greater contributor) to successfully raising two happy, healthy children.

Michael Roland Walker and I were married in 1980, when I was beginning graduate school. Our marriage was actually our second shot at getting it right, as we had dated briefly one summer when I was home from college. That summer, by nights I worked as a waitress, and by day I was at the pool, tanning and playing water volleyball (my favorite sport, as it is the only one I know of that is improved by playing with a drink in one hand). Mike and I met at the pool and enjoyed each other's company, but we both had other interests (i.e., other girlfriends and boyfriends); thus, when the summer ended, so did our relationship. After graduation, my first job, as a microbiologist working in quality control in the food industry, brought me back to Dallas.

Although I loved my job, taking direction from others has never been my strong suit (this trait is hereditary). I soon realized that without a Ph.D., achieving professionally the type of independence I took for granted in every other aspect of my life would be problematic. So I tested the waters by taking graduate classes at night, and I found that I got A's easily and enjoyed being back in school. These grades and a reasonable (but not stellar) GRE score were enough to gain me admission (without a stipend) to the Ph.D. biology program at The University of Texas-Dallas. During this time, Mike and I became reacquainted when we fortuitously bumped into each other while clubbing one night in Dallas (another activity I had gravitated to because it was improved with drink in hand). One date led to another and, after a two-year romance, we married in 1980. It was during this period that the graduate school at UT-Dallas and I had a "falling out" when they tried to coerce me into taking a class I was not interested in just so there would be enough students to "make" the class for a professor who needed the teaching credit. This ruffled my independent spirit, so I re-took the GRE exam and obtained a higher score that qualified me for the graduate program at UT Southwestern Medical School. Armed with that score and a track record of A's in graduate-level courses, I transferred to the Ph.D. program in the Cell Biology department at UT Southwestern.

Graduate school was relatively uneventful until 1983, when our daughter Ashley was born. At the time, I had passed my qualifying exams and was in the home stretch of completing my dissertation in the laboratory of Dr. Jerry Shay. Interestingly, Jerry had been a postdoc in the MCD Biology department at the University of Colorado while I was an undergraduate there, and I had narrowly missed doing my undergraduate research project with his group. Jerry was an inspiring thesis advisor, and I still marvel at his enthusiasm and vision for his research. He and the other faculty were supportive during my pregnancy, and I was able to return to the lab quickly after Ashley was born (we found good daycare for her in a private home). As I recall, the latency period for the tumor cells I had injected into nude mice for the final series of experiments for my thesis (just prior to going into labor) was exactly the same duration as my maternity leave. Upon my return, I sacrificed the mice, took the tumor counts, and demonstrated that we had epigenetically modified tumorigenicity to complete my thesis project.

By the time our second child, Christopher, was born in 1987, we were in North Carolina, where I was a staff fellow at the National Institute of Environmental Health Sciences (NIEHS), and by this time we had become all too familiar with the obstacles associated with finding good daycare. Prior to having our second child, I had begun to work with others at the Institute and the Environmental Protection Agency (EPA) to get approval for an onsite daycare center for NIEHS and EPA employees on the NIEHS campus in Research Triangle Park. The process took about two years, but we were ultimately successful. The First Environments Child Care Center opened at NIEHS in 1986, and I was the first president of the parent-run Board of Directors. NIEHS provided the space and underwrote much of the budget for the center. The parents' organization provided oversight for the center; hired the first director and assisted her with staff hiring; worked out a plan to partner with the NIEHS cafeteria to provide food service; scavenged garage sales for toys, linens and other supplies; and provided much of the infrastructure, including playground equipment, cribs, etc., to open the center on a shoestring budget. The daycare center was a huge success, both financially and in terms of the exceptional high-quality care it provided to children of NIEHS and EPA employees. To this day, the center remains a source of pride for the Institute, the EPA and, truth be told, for me as well.

With the availability of top-notch daycare at First Environments, I returned to work soon after Chris' birth, bringing him to work with me. Ashley was also briefly at the daycare center until she started kindergarten the following fall. Besides knowing that my children were receiving excellent care, I also enjoyed being with them as I went to and from work each day. However, the disadvantage was the "daycare dash" that occurred at 5 o'clock each afternoon, when I had to pause my experiments and run to get the kids from daycare. Chris remained at the First Environments until he was about 4, even after I had left NIEHS to take my first position as a principal investigator at the Chemical Industry Institute of Toxicology, also in Research Triangle Park. Soon, however, I began to travel professionally, and it was quite difficult for Mike to make the long drive to and from home to the daycare center twice a day when I was away. We were sad to withdraw Chris from First Environments but, happily, were able to place him in a good Montessori program until he entered kindergarten.

Since Chris and Ashley were now both in Raleigh and I was commuting to Research Triangle Park, Mike became the primary go-to person whenever the kids were sick or needed to be home from school. This relieved me of the responsibility but, of course, meant that he was now shouldering the vast majority of the day-to-day care of our children. He did this with aplomb and, as it turns out, he was equipped with the patience I lacked when it came to working through homework meltdowns or dealing with routine discipline issues. Thus, he was — and continues to be — a wonderful father and role model for our children.

In time, our children entered the public school system, and we were fortunate to live in excellent school districts that provided them with first-rate educations that prepared them well for entering college. It was during this time that I was recruited back to Texas in 1992 to join the faculty in the Department of Carcinogenesis at M. D. Anderson's Science Park-Research Division. We were delighted to return "home" to Texas, and the Department of Carcinogenesis was the perfect academic home for my developing research program. I was fortunate enough to come to M. D. Anderson as an associate professor, and I became tenured shortly thereafter, when I received my first R01 grant.

The environment at M. D. Anderson was incredibly fertile for growing a successful research program, and relatively rapidly I was running one of the larger research programs in the department, was promoted to full professor, and eventually received an endowed professorship. Interacting with my colleagues in the department and on the main campus as well as outside the institution has been one of the great joys of my career. In fact, the fantastic research environment and the incredible faculty at M. D. Anderson are two of the main reasons that I have stayed here for the past 16 years despite numerous, and often tempting, offers to relocate my research program. In addition, both the institution and my department chair have been very supportive of my many extramural activities, where I have the opportunity to represent M. D. Anderson on the national and international level and which over the years have become quite substantial. These activities have included numerous advisory board appointments within the NIH, at several universities, and with patient advocacy groups focused on diseases related to my research program. I have also had the opportunity to be very involved in the American Association for Cancer Research and the Society of Toxicology and have been elected to the presidential chain of the Society of Toxicology, for which I will serve as president in 2009.

People who know my hectic schedule will sometimes ask me how I managed to raise a family. I usually quip that I did it by "giving up being an interesting person." Of course, this is said tongue-in-cheek, but it *is* true that once the children were older and in school, our lives outside of work held little time for activities beyond family, school and church. Although we didn't always have dinner on the table at the same time every evening (*there's* an understatement), when we were at the table, we talked rather than watched TV. I can truthfully say that we never missed a play, parent teacher conference or ballgame with our children. The scheduling required to accomplish this was challenging to say the least. Fortunately, the escalation of my professional demands coincided with the kids' graduating from high school and leaving for college, and, as an empty nester, it became easier for me to meet my ever-increasing professional responsibilities. As an added bonus, with the kids on their own, I now have time to become "an interesting person" again. As a start, I received my open water scuba diving certification last fall (at age 52) and did my first blue water dive in the Caribbean last winter.

Most parents question their parenting skills, and I, too, have worried about whether I have given enough to my children considering all the demands of my career. Fortunately, both our children have grown to be wonderful adults, leaving little room for second guessing. And, as my daughter volunteered one day, "There are worse things in life than to have a successful mom as a role model." Bless you, Ashley and Chris, and, most of all, thank you, Mike.

Dihua Yu, M.D., Ph.D.

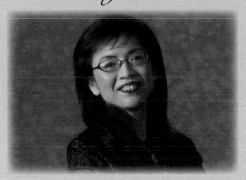

**Professor of Molecular and Cellular Oncology
Nylene Eckles Distinguished Professorship
in Breast Cancer Research**

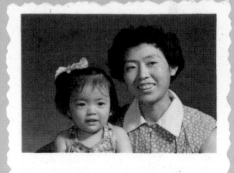

Dihua was 15 months old when this photo was taken with her mother, Renping Yang.

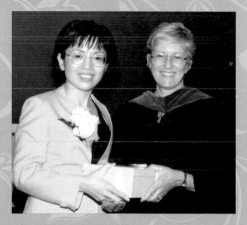

Sizzling temperatures were part of Dihua's introduction to Houston and her Ph.D. training at The University of Texas Graduate School of Biomedical Sciences in 1986.

Dihua received the E. N. Cobb Faculty Scholar Award from Margaret Kripke, Ph.D., at M.D. Anderson's Faculty Honors Convocation in 2000.

was born into a physicians' family. Both of my parents are medical doctors. My father is the fifth generation of doctors in the Yu family, and my grandfather on my mother's side was the Chief Physician for General Zhang Xue-Liang in the 1930s. Not surprisingly, my parents expected me to be a physician. When I was in elementary school, my father told me that he and the previous generations of Yu family physicians had all published books, recording their specialties and experiences in dealing with very challenging patient cases. He told me that he expected to see my book when I grew up. I am glad that I did not disappoint him, and I recently gave him a new book that I had edited.

My mother was my role model as a career woman. She devoted herself to her patients and her family. She gave all her time, energy and resources to others and left almost nothing for herself. She was the chair of the Department of Internal Medicine at a more than 3,000-employee hospital in Beijing and frequently had to take care of over 80 patients a day in the clinic. Meanwhile, she managed to do almost everything for her three children (without much help from my father) so that we could concentrate on our studies. I still cannot figure out how she did it. She began teaching me three Chinese characters every day when I was 3 years of age; this equipped me with a middle-school-level reading ability when I entered the first grade. During my teenage years, my mother told me: "Dihua, external beauty can fade away as one gets old no matter how hard you try to keep it; on the other hand, the beauty inside a person — for example, a loving heart and a broad knowledge — can be kept and grows more as one ages and can be passed to future generations." Her wisdom has guided my life.

I was "a nerd" in school. I was given nicknames by other students for receiving perfect test scores (100 percent) in every subject. I loved to read all kinds of books. In addition to Chinese and foreign literature, history, philosophy and poems, I also enjoyed reading about Newton, Darwin, Copernicus, Galileo and Einstein. I was most fascinated and touched by the story of Madame Curie — I admired her and wanted to follow in her footsteps. I decided that I would not be the sixth generation of physicians in the Yu family and instead chose to study chemistry at Beijing University when I applied for college. However, my father believed that I would have a great future as a physician. He talked to the principal of my high school, who was a patient of his, and without consulting me, changed my college choice to study medicine at the Capital Medical University.

Thus, I unwillingly started my medical school training in 1978. Although I was a straight-A student in medical school, I did not enjoy the courses very much, as they mostly required memorizing descriptive, known facts. I was always more intrigued by novel scientific findings and was eager to know the unknown. However, I began to appreciate my medical education after I started my internship in a hospital in Beijing. When we were making morning rounds, the patients would eagerly look at us to assess their diseases and trusted us with their lives. I started to understand why my parents loved their profession and why they were so dedicated to their patients. It was rewarding that I was able to help some patients. But there were also cases in which I felt helpless and powerless. I remember one instance of a young woman of my age who had colon cancer with liver metastasis and died right in front of me even with intensive care. We tried every treatment available in the 1980s but were unable to save her life. I was sad and disappointed that we physicians had such limited tools to deal with aggressive diseases.

This and several other similar incidents made me feel that medicine as an academic discipline was quite primitive and relied mostly on descriptive and correlative knowledge. I thought that we needed a better understanding of diseases and more effective medicines based on that understanding. This motivated me to go back to graduate school. Since I had developed an interest in understanding how the brain functions in human diseases, I entered an M.S. program in 1983, right after graduation from medical school, to study neuro-cardiophysiology (there was no Ph.D. program in China at that time). My mentor was Professor Zengfu Liu, from whom I learned not only how to address scientific questions related to a specific research project but also some general principles of conducting research. However, the research environment in China at that time was not favorable, and I frequently became very frustrated due to the lack of key reagents and needed equipment and to the difficulty of obtaining the most recent publications. Fortunately, after Richard Nixon's visit to China in the 1970s, the Chinese government initiated in the 1980s an "open door" policy that brought unprecedented changes. It became possible for us to study abroad and to learn from the best in an outstanding environment.

I came to the United States in the summer of 1986 and began my Ph.D. training at the Graduate School of Biomedical Sciences (GSBS) at The University of Texas Health Science Center in Houston. I first joined a protein chemistry lab in the UT Medical School for my thesis study. My mentor asked me to learn molecular cloning through tutorials under two newly recruited faculty, outstanding molecular biologists from Stanford University (Dr. David Loose) and MIT (Dr. Mien-Chie Hung). After 20 months of very challenging learning and hard work, I successfully cloned the full-length cDNA for a calmodulin-binding protein. However, my mentor then asked me to pass the cDNA clone to a postdoctoral fellow in the lab for functional study and assigned me to clone another gene. This meant that I had to start my thesis research all over again as a third-year graduate student! I share this experience because things like this can happen to anyone, and, when they do, you just need to find a way to move on. I expressed my frustration to the GSBS student advisor, Ms. Gaughan. Fortunately, the GSBS has a good tradition of protecting students, and I was advised to move to a different lab for my thesis study.

In October 1988, I joined Dr. Mien-Chie Hung's laboratory at M. D. Anderson Cancer Center for my Ph.D. thesis research. Mien-Chie is one of the hardest-working scientists I know, and his love of research is contagious! He always challenged us to ask important questions and to think outside the current dogma. I was inspired by him to clone the tumor growth factor-beta receptor so that we could study its function in human cancer, and to study transcriptional regulation of the HER2/ErbB2/neu oncogene so that we could identify a new approach to turn off the oncogene. I truly enjoyed learning state-of-the-art molecular biology techniques and making new discoveries. Interestingly, my research project studying the regulation and function of the HER2/ErbB2 oncogene provided me with opportunities not only to learn the fundamental approaches of basic science but also to link basic research back to medicine. Specifically, my thesis research revealed that the adenovirus E1A gene transcriptionally represses the HER2/neu gene and inhibits HER2/neu-induced transformation, tumorigenesis, and metastasis. Based on my findings and on additional research by other trainees along the same lines, M. D. Anderson and several other institutions performed clinical trials using E1A to treat HER2-positive cancer patients and demonstrated some clinical efficacy. This gave me a rewarding feeling, similar to what I had experienced while I was doing my internship. It also made me realize that by asking clinically important questions, I as a scientist also could have the opportunity to help many patients, as my parents had always wanted me to do.

Another important part of my thesis research was to study the oncogenic function of HER2/neu. Since the first patient whose death I had witnessed died of cancer metastasis and since M. D. Anderson has an outstanding environment for studying cancer metastasis, I initiated an investigation of whether HER2/neu promotes cancer metastasis using a defined experimental system rather than a correlative study. I clearly demonstrated that overexpression of HER2/neu induced higher metastatic potential in cancer cells. Back in the early 1990s, metastasis research was done mostly at the general biology or cell biology level. I, on the other hand, was able to apply molecular approaches for understanding mechanisms of cancer metastasis because of my molecular biology training from Mien-Chie and the cancer biology expertise at M. D. Anderson. This provided me with a unique opportunity when Dr. Suresh Mohla at the National Cancer Institute (NCI) initiated an R03 grant mechanism to solicit proposals using molecular biology approaches to study cancer metastasis. I submitted an R03 proposal with my medical degree while I was still a GSBS student.

In April 1991, I was informed that my R03 application had received a top score and would be one of the 10 proposals nationwide to be funded by R03 grants. Before I was notified about the R03 grant in early 1991, I had also applied for a postdoctoral position in the lab of Dr. Bert Vogelstein, who had been named by the journal *Science* as scientist of the year in 1990. At about the same time I received the grant notice, I also got a handwritten letter from Dr. Vogelstein telling me that he had an opening for my postdoctoral training in his laboratory in the summer of 1991. My career was at a crossroads! I was debating whether to stay at M. D. Anderson to carry out the research in the funded R03 grant or to move to Johns Hopkins for postdoctoral training with Dr. Vogelstein. I had several discussions with Mien-Chie and with Dr. Garth Nicolson, who was the chair of the Department of Tumor Biology at that time. Garth said that he could not understand why I was even considering giving up the incoming grant to be a postdoctoral fellow. He then promised to promote me to instructor right away and to assign me a lab space if I stayed at M. D. Anderson, but I was still having difficulty making my decision.

Then, I found that I was pregnant with my first child, and that coming event convinced me to stay at M. D. Anderson, as I was sure I could succeed in carrying out the research proposed in the R03 grant in this nurturing and friendly environment even while pregnant. I was awarded the R03 NIH grant in July 1991, three months after I graduated from the Ph.D. program. That year, the NIH funding rate was at a historically low point and it was very difficult to obtain grants, even for established investigators. My success in obtaining the R03 was partially due to my exposure to grant writing while I was a graduate student, as I had always worked with Mien-Chie when he was submitting his grant applications. I share this experience with students and postdoctoral fellows to let them know that assisting your mentor can better equip you for future career challenges. In September 1991, I was given the junior faculty title of instructor and was assigned two benches at M. D. Anderson. I will never know whether I made the best decision.

Pursuing the R03 grant allowed me to publish four first-authored papers, but it also generated more scientific questions. Therefore, I decided to apply for an R29 grant in 1992. As I was actively writing the grant application, I had a chance to meet an invited speaker, who was a distinguished senior scientist. When he heard that I was writing an R29 proposal, he told me, "My advice is don't waste your time. Reviewers are not going to give a five-year NIH grant to an instructor, especially in the current funding environment." As you can imagine, this was a very discouraging message. But, I told myself, "My chance is zero if I do not apply, but my opportunity will be greater than zero if I do apply." So I made substantial efforts to prepare the R29 proposal, and the application was reviewed by the Path B

Study Section. To this day, I am very grateful that the reviewers of that study section gave me outstanding and constructive suggestions. I revised one cycle and received the funding notification in 1993.

After this, I started to look for a tenure-track assistant professorship to obtain an opportunity for an independent research career. At that time, the Department of Tumor Biology at M. D. Anderson had such an opening, so I applied for it. After a couple of months, Garth Nicolson, the department chair, told me that he had had a faculty meeting to discuss my application and that most of the faculty had supported it but one had said "I don't think she is ready." Garth told me that it would be very difficult to have a smooth start to such a challenging career with an opponent in the same department. He said, however, that there were many other opportunities at the institution: for example, Dr. Raphael Pollock in the Department of Surgical Oncology was recruiting for a tenure-track assistant professor. Garth told me that if I were interested, he would be happy to pass my CV on.

Within a few days, Raphael contacted me about the available position in Surgical Oncology, and we had a very nice conversation. He told me that he had received more than 80 CVs for the position and was most impressed by mine, especially by my grant funding. He wanted to offer me the position and bring it to upper-level leaders for approval. However, I had something else in my mind. I told him that because a colleague at the institution thought that I was not ready for a tenure-track assistant professorship, I needed to prove my credentials to my colleagues *and* to myself. Thus, I did not want to accept his offer right away but first wanted to seriously look for a tenure-track assistant professor position outside the institution. I would only take the M. D. Anderson offer after I had a written offer from outside. I am thankful that Raphael was so understanding and supportive. He agreed to my proposal and said he would hold the position for me. I sent application letters to 12 universities/institutes for tenure-track assistant professor positions and was invited for an interview by seven. After I had received three offers, I declined the other invitations. I then brought the written offers back to Raphael and asked him to put them into my file. I told him that in the future, should anyone question my qualifications for a tenure-track position at M. D. Anderson, he could show them these written offers.

Raphael and I began scientific collaborations in January 1994. I ran my breast cancer research lab and, in addition, Raphael asked me to help build a sarcoma research lab with him. My parents had always told me that, by strengthening my boss's position, I was strengthening my own position as well. I therefore put my heart and soul into leading those two research groups. I provided daily guidance to students, postdoctoral fellows and research assistants in both labs. We published many high-quality papers and received multiple NIH and Department of Defense (DOD) grants. Several faculty inquired how I could successfully manage to run two labs that had different research focuses while many faculty were stressed by running one lab with one general research direction. They asked, "What is your secret?" But there was no secret! I worked about 100 hours a week and did not take a single day of vacation in 13 years. Although I have now moved to the Department of Molecular and Cellular Oncology, I am positive that those 13 years of hard work allowed me to build a solid scientific base and taught me leadership. My career rapidly advanced from junior faculty to my current established status because of the quick accumulation of knowledge, experience, leadership skills, and success in research, education and service to the scientific community that were the direct result of working very hard. Just as my Mom had told me when I was a teenager, the skills and knowledge within me had accumulated and grown. Working closely with Raphael, I also learned some of his techniques for handling sensitive issues. In some cases, these were eye-opening experiences that allowed me to gain some measure of political wisdom.

I also have been very fortunate to have Mien-Chie as my mentor even after I began my independent research career. Mien-Chie and I have regular meetings and discussions. He sets very high standards in research, education and services. These have been my career challenges. Whenever colleagues and friends told me "You work too hard," I smiled and told them that I knew another person who worked even harder, and I meant Mien-Chie. Inspired by him, I tell myself "We only have this life once, so we should do something important with it." Because of my medical background, I identified translational research as my focus. I want to use research approaches to answer and address clinically important questions. For example, our studies on the mechanisms of Herceptin resistance revealed that loss of PTEN rendered breast cancers resistant to Herceptin. We then developed combination therapy strategies that allow us to overcome Herceptin resistance mediated by PTEN loss. This has led to a phase I/II clinical trial, and it has been really rewarding to see that about half the patients on the trial have benefited from this newly developed strategy. Our work has also been recognized by the scientific community: in a commentary in *Nature News,* in the *New England Journal of Medicine*, and in a 2006 *Science* article by the previous NIH director, Dr. Harold Varmus, reviewing 50 years of progress in developing anticancer therapies.

As far as my personal life, I guess the younger generation would consider my current lifestyle "boring." I was an amateur dancer in elementary and middle school (and occasionally in medical school and graduate school in China). In high school and beyond in China, I spent my weekends visiting art galleries, attending concerts or going to theatre shows. I got married when I was a graduate student in China. My husband, Ping, majored in electrical engineering as an undergraduate and in graduate school at Rice University. He supports me and takes a major share of our family responsibilities. As mentioned previously, I was pregnant with my first child in 1991, when I was the principal investigator on the funded R03 grant. I did not take a single day off during pregnancy and I did not stop bench work. I returned to work in blue jeans 12 days after my son was born, and I attended a local scientific meeting. At the meeting, I won first prize for a poster presentation, an award that provided me with full travel support to an international meeting in Singapore.

In 1998, when I was in the eighth month of pregnancy with my daughter, my lab and Raphael's lab were scheduled to move from the Yellow Zone to the newly built Tan Zone lab space. As the lab head, I organized all elements of the move for the two labs without taking any of Raphael's time. After one week of intensive moving, we pretty much settled into our new location. Before I went home that evening, I took a final tour of the new lab and was relieved that the move had gone smoothly. However, when I returned to my office, suddenly my water broke. Since I was only eight months pregnant, I had not yet arranged for transportation to the hospital. My husband was an hour's drive away from M. D. Anderson, and I did not want to risk having the baby in my office, so I walked quietly and slowly to Garage 5 to drive myself to the Woman's Hospital of Texas. Fortunately, in the garage I met Mien-Chie, who was on his way to dinner with several faculty friends. Seeing my situation, he postponed the dinner and dropped me at the hospital building entrance. I took an elevator upstairs to the delivery room and had my daughter at 1:30 a.m. on August 8, 1988. At 10 a.m. that day, I called the lab to tell them that my daughter had been born early and that I wouldn't be able to make the 10:30 a.m. meeting that I had originally scheduled to discuss revision of a manuscript for *Molecular Cell*. I came back to work two weeks later, led the team effort to finalize the revision, and submitted the revised manuscript before the deadline. The paper was accepted for publication soon afterward.

I have to say that it is not easy to juggle personal and professional demands, but I am fortunate to have a supportive family. Three days before I delivered my son, my mother flew from Beijing to Houston to help me. She had just had a mastectomy after being diagnosed with node-positive breast cancer. Although she could not even lift her left arm then, she insisted on taking care of my son so that I could sleep through the night and go work the next day fully energized. Later, her breast cancer progressed with lung metastases and she had a second surgery. A few years later, she had bone and brain metastasis. While she was hospitalized in Beijing, I had a few opportunities to speak at scientific meetings in China and got to visit her. I could tell from her eyes that she was very happy to see me. However, she would always say, "You should go back. I don't want you to slow down your work for me." My mother had a big loving heart and was totally selfless. After she left Houston, my in-laws came here. They have given their love and care to my children, allowing me to better concentrate on my work. Meanwhile, I did find a way to be with my children while working. I began to bring my son to work with me on weekends when he was 2 years old. We would bring computer games or fun toys, and, while he played, I would talk with colleagues and lab members. Then, we would go to the cafeteria and have a baked potato, one of my son's favorite foods. Amazingly, coming to work with Mom on weekends became a real treat for him. After he entered middle school, I began bringing my daughter to work on some weekends, and she also very much enjoys this routine. Although I sometimes feel guilty for not spending enough time with my children, they seem to understand and are both good students who hold high academic standards themselves. Some people ask what I do during my free time. I do not have much free time, but I do find time to read. Reading gives me peace of mind, enjoyment and keeps me young at heart. I also go to the gym to run on the treadmill on Saturdays and Sundays. At this stage of my career, I also have many opportunities to travel around the world, which not only meets my professional needs but also enriches my personal experience.

Although biomedical research is challenging and demanding, it can be really rewarding. I feel that I have one of the best jobs in the world. I once told my children that I wouldn't trade jobs with President Bush, and I meant it. My profession allows me to learn new things and make new discoveries every day. Our research brings new diagnostic tools and novel therapeutics to benefit patients. As an educator, I have the unique pleasure of bringing up a younger generation of scientists. I have a typical "Chinese Mom" mentality in that I have a high expectation for my trainees and care about them as if they were my children. When my trainees show progress in their studies and receive awards, I am as happy and proud as when I get straight-A report cards and award plaques from my children. I enjoy doing research and also cherish my ability to provide younger scientists with needed help. I am fortunate that my dream of following Madame Curie's path in research has partially come true. My research and education efforts are having an impact on patients' lives and on young peoples' careers, and this gives me a rewarding sense of achievement that cannot be measured by money or fame. Whenever I meet young people who demonstrate a true love of research, I naturally want to pass along my knowledge and experience to help them succeed. For those young people who share my dream, I have a few special, specific pieces of advice. First, it is important to have a clear vision and a clear career goal and to persistently work toward it without distractions. I have had some trainees who were very bright with great potential but who were easily distracted and did not use their time wisely. Second, as a scientist and researcher, one needs to be resilient and remain optimistic. Experimentation can frequently fail and requires searching for the correct answers/approaches again and again. I have seen trainees get depressed when their experiments do not work and then stop pursuing the solutions. Unfortunately, this will never lead one out of a bad cycle. Handling failure with a positive mindset leads to final success, which will be even more rewarding. Third, find a good mentor who can guide you and inspire you to develop a successful biomedical research career. I am very fortunate to have Dr. Mien-Chie Hung as my mentor. More recently, Dr. Margaret Kripke has given me critical career advice and shared her wisdom on leadership with me. She encouraged me to participate in the Faculty Leadership Academy, where I learned to take a balanced approach when handling conflict rather than the avoidance or compromise approaches I was used to taking. As a high-achieving woman scientist and a senior woman faculty leader, Dr. Kripke is an important role model for me.

Currently, I have two important professional missions. First, I want to perform high-quality cancer research that will impact patient care. Second, I want to provide leadership and serve as an active educator to bring up the younger generation of scientists so that they will be ready to continue the fight against cancer and succeed in their careers. I enjoy working with my colleagues and trainees who share my vision and passion in fulfilling these missions. The daily opportunity to interact with bright people who have enthusiastic minds is a precious gift. Life is good.

Epilogue

Soon after joining The University of Texas M. D. Anderson Cancer Center as Provost and Executive Vice President, I was delighted to discover that the institution had launched a formal effort focused on the recruitment, retention and development of women faculty. Elizabeth Travis, Ph.D., who prior to my arrival was appointed by Margaret Kripke, Ph.D., leads the new Office of Women Faculty Programs, which is dedicated to the advancement of women faculty and the establishment of M. D. Anderson as an international leader in offering exciting opportunities for women physicians and scientists.

Much of M. D. Anderson's recent progress in cancer research, patient care, education and prevention has been possible because of Margaret's contributions over more than two decades. Not only has she blazed a trail for other women to follow, but she also has inspired substantial improvements to help all faculty. For example, she influenced the creation of an academic leadership academy for faculty training, she instituted a rigorous laboratory review process for each of our laboratory investigators and she established periodic external reviews of all basic science departments. In addition to serving as the first female faculty member selected for top management at M. D. Anderson, she has worked tirelessly during two terms on the three-member President's Cancer Panel to advance national strategies to control cancer.

The Office of Women Faculty Programs is especially meaningful to me because I have strongly supported development of women's careers in academic medicine and understand very well the impact of this initiative. I came to M. D. Anderson from the Vanderbilt-Ingram Cancer Center in Tennessee, an institution where about half of the basic science department chairs are women and where the leadership team is fairly balanced in its gender mix. That diversity, which served Vanderbilt well, certainly is a key component for the continuing success of M. D. Anderson. I am extremely proud that Jennifer Pietenpol, Ph.D., who served as my research director, has recently been named Director of the Vanderbilt-Ingram Cancer Center. Supporting and advancing the careers of women faculty is a vital issue at all academic medical institutions, where women still tend to remain under-represented on the faculty and more heavily concentrated at entry level ranks. A few years ago, Eric Neilson, M.D., Chairman of Medicine at Vanderbilt University Medical School, published a collection of stories about women faculty at Vanderbilt, and it was very well received. When Liz Travis told me about plans to develop a similar book at M. D. Anderson, I enthusiastically encouraged her efforts.

Two women, in particular, have had influential roles in helping me achieve my own research success. Bettie Sue Masters, Ph.D., now at The University of Texas Health Science Center in San Antonio, served on my dissertation committee when I was at The University of Texas Southwestern Medical School in Dallas and provided valuable advice and guidance while I received my graduate training. Terri Stadtman, Ph.D., my research mentor for a National Institutes of Health summer fellowship that I completed as a medical student, has been another key influence for me. In fact, without her positive recommendation, I doubt that I would have been selected later for a postdoctoral fellowship and Howard Hughes Research Associate position in the laboratory of Nobel Laureate Daniel Nathans, M.D., at Johns Hopkins Medical School. The importance of these and so many other women as teachers, mentors, coaches and friends cannot be overstated.

The engaging stories shared in *Legends and Legacies* prove that the path to accomplished academic careers is not always direct and there may be many pitfalls along the way. One common thread among the authors is their desire and drive for success. As we look to the future in an increasingly fast-paced environment, all physicians and scientists — both men and women — will need even stronger mentoring and support for career development, which means that those already established in their fields must make time to pass along valuable experiences and advice to those just beginning to plan careers in academic medicine. I believe the personal journeys of the women faculty included in this book will help inspire others to provide such crucial mentoring.

Of course, it must be noted that over the past century women have made some of the most significant contributions in the arenas of science and medicine. Among early pioneers are Rosalind Franklin, a gifted scientist whose X-ray data on the structure of DNA laid the foundation for Watson and Crick's research; and Marie Curie, world-renowned physicist, discoverer of radium and Nobel Prize winner for her work in the fields of physics and chemistry. The achievements of these women are valued not so much because women made them, but because gifted scientists who happened to be women overcame obstacles and were ultimately judged by their contributions rather than their gender. This is as it should be.

Concerning the role of women in the development of M. D. Anderson, it is obvious from reading Texas history books that Frances Goff (born in 1916 in Kenedy, Texas) had a remarkable role. Frances was neither a scientist nor a clinician, but she was truly devoted to assuring the success of M. D. Anderson. From 1937 to 1944, she served in several positions with the

Texas House of Representatives, State Senate, the Office of the Governor and the Texas Railroad Commission. After a stint in the military (1944 to 1946) during World War II, she then worked for Governor Allan Shivers for five years. In 1951, she joined the staff of R. Lee Clark, M.D., who was President of M. D. Anderson, and she had a pivotal role in obtaining state funding to build our initial hospital, which opened in 1954 in the Texas Medical Center. She helped direct fundraising, planning and construction of what would ultimately become the most comprehensive cancer center in the world. Of relevance to the topic of this book, Ms. Goff also served from 1952 to 1994 as director of the American Legion Auxiliary Bluebonnet Girls State that each summer gave young women from throughout Texas opportunities to learn about government and how to become future leaders. Among highly accomplished leaders who emerged from the Girls State program was Ann Richards, who eventually was elected state treasurer and governor of Texas. In 1965, Ms. Goff invited the first black woman, Barbara Jordan, who then was a state senator, to speak at Girls State, thereby opening opportunities for young African-American women to participate in Girls State.

The career paths of women pioneers in science, as well as many of the women celebrated in this book, were often convoluted and contained few signposts. With the insights, guidance and mentoring offered by the women who share their stories here — and by others like them — future generations of women in academic medicine hopefully will have smoother journeys. We must discard past gender stereotypes and do everything possible to attract, train and support the best and brightest minds to meet the challenges of conquering such relentless and stubborn problems as cancer. Future generations are counting on all of us.

Raymond N. DuBois, M.D., Ph.D.
Provost and Executive Vice President
Professor of Gastrointestinal Medical Oncology
The University of Texas M. D. Anderson Cancer Center